Doin' it With the Lights On

Exploits of a Paramedic

For permissions, bulk ordering, or speaking engagements
contact the author at: www.JRStine.com

Published in collaboration with
Season Press and Fortitude Graphic Design and Printing
Design and layout by Sean Hollins-Fortitude Graphic Design
Cover and author photo by Greg Wardecke

Library of Congress Control Number: 2015936650

Stine, James R. Jr.
Doin' it with the Lights On: Exploits of a Paramedic- Non-fiction
p.cm
1. James R. Stine-Biography 2. Medical-Paramedics
3. Medical-Social Issues 4. Medical-Politics

ISBN-10: 0-9863173-4-9
ISBN-13: 978-0-9863173-4-7

Printed in the United States of America

FIRST EDITION
10 9 8 7 6 5 4 3 2 1

*To my parents, Jim and Jeanette, who
provided me with everything I needed…and luckily
for me only half of what I wanted.*

J.S.

TABLE OF CONTENTS

PROLOGUE

What you are about to read is a no-holds barred account of a career in Emergency Medical Services (EMS) that began in 1977, and continues as of this publication. It is brutally honest in its candor and content. It is anything but politically correct. It speaks to the human condition that, being under tremendous stress can bring out the very best—or very worst in people.

Although Hollywood has made attempts to showcase the world in which paramedics and EMT's work, most of those attempts are unrealistic; being either vanilla in nature or over dramatized. Through it all, EMS remains the largely overlooked leg of the emergency triad. Together, the police and fire departments represent the other two legs, and have been in existence since our country's inception. Modern EMS has been in existence far less than fifty years.

In this book, I will give you a small taste of what it is really like to be a part of modern EMS. If you are one of the vast majorities that know very little about EMS and are in no way connected to this business, I want you to know that every word contained here is true. The people, places, and events that you will read about are real and absolutely authentic.

At the guidance of legal counsel, the names and any personal identifying information in regards to HIPAA (Health Insurance Portability and Accountability Act) statutes have been changed to protect the privacy of the subjects. Each quote is accurate and in proper context of the story or incident being told. The opinions put forth are mine alone.

If you have just a passing interest, or if you are contemplating a career choice in this field, these true and factual stories and events will give you an accurate look at the life of an emergency pre-hospital health care provider. Regardless of the reasons for selecting this book, it is what this business is all about, from someone who has lived it for more than thirty-five years.

What exactly is EMS, and who are the people who work in this field of public health and emergency service? How and what do they think in regards to the functions and performances of their duties? How extensive is their training and what are their responsibilities? How does EMS fit in, and interact with area police and fire departments, as well as hospital-based personnel?

The chapters that follow will answer these questions and more. The experiences told here range from the gratifying and near heroic ambulance calls, to calls that elicit tears of anger, profound disgust, and sadness. Some may find what I share somewhat insensitive and perhaps even offensive.

But through it all, I am most confident that you will come to know and understand the few who do a job that most people can't even imagine performing. Many times they are doin' it under tremendous stress. They are doin' it with remarkable intensity and concentration. Finally, when it really matters, when the patient's outcome is in doubt, you'll find that there are EMT's and paramedics pulling out all the stops—working hard and *Doin' It With The Lights On!*

Doin' it With the Lights On

Exploits of a Paramedic

James R. Stine Jr.

Season Press

Chapter 1
Starting With Roy and Johnny

The phone rings and it instantly awakens me. As I momentarily fumble for the phone in the dark station, I answer it to the voice of our dispatcher. She quickly tells me that a woman has just given birth to a full-term baby...in the middle of her front yard.

It is 7 a.m., and I had already been on duty for almost twenty-three hours, and my co-worker Bob Ristau and I, had a little more than an hour to go before completing our usual twenty-four hour shift. The shift had already been grueling, and we looked forward to one last hour of peace before handing over the reins to the next crew. Now, that was going to be later than usual.

As the dispatcher gave us the address and some of the other pertinent information, I was thinking, *Oh man, this could be nothing but trouble.* I replied to the dispatcher (who was verbally excited about the whole situation) that we were on our way.

"We have a newborn lying in the grass at someone's house," I said to Bob who was now awake and getting dressed.

"What in the heck does that mean?" he said, as he tried to make sense out of what I was saying.

"Who knows? It doesn't sound right to me either, but the dispatcher said there is a woman that just gave birth in her front yard. The address is out on a distant country road several minutes away. I guess the baby couldn't wait another hour until we were relieved by the next crew." As I thought about it, I'd yet to meet a newborn that could tell time anyway.

As we scrambled out of our south station and jumped into our ambulance, we notified our dispatcher that we were en route, double-checked the address, and flipped on our lights and siren. Nearly three miles into our trip, I mentioned to Bob how nicely the cars were cooperating by getting out of our way. That was the wrong thing to say. Suddenly, nothing would ever be the same.

While driving on a two-lane highway headed into a small town called Berrien Springs, a full-size van, that was immediately in front of us, pulled to the right to reveal a small car in front of them that was moving slower than anticipated. As the two-lane road expanded into four lanes, I thought in milliseconds, *Okay, I'm going to move to his left since he is supposed to move to the right and come to a stop...wait...what's he doing? He's still in front of me... not pulling over... I see no brake lights... Holy Christ, he just flipped his left turn signal on and he's still in front of me...He's turning hard to his left...this is going to be bad!*

As I skidded to the left, his turn signal blinked twice as he pulled hard directly in the pathway of my ambulance. BANG! I hit him in the left-rear fender. The rear windshield on his hatchback exploded, and suddenly the whole world was ablaze with sparkling and multi-colored glass. For half a second, that's all either Bob or I could see.

The ambulance ricocheted off the car, and I instantly looked into my side view mirror to see the little car rolling over and off the highway into a large yard. Dirt and sod were thrown high into the air and the car appeared to be coming apart. I struggled to bring the ambulance under control and to a stop. All that ran through my mind was, *Why did he pull in front of me? Didn't he hear or see me? Where were his damn brake lights? Dear God, was I at fault? Was I going too fast? Did I drive with due regard? How many people were in the car?*

As we came to a stop, Bob had already notified our dispatch center that we were involved in a horrendous accident, and to send help. When we stopped, we hit the pavement running. It only took us a few short seconds to reach the site of where the car came to rest.

We found a man, who appeared to be in his late twenties, unconscious in the car. A youngster about five-years-old was laying in the grass along side the road. He had no pulse. Neither of them had been wearing seat belts and there was no car seat for the child. I was absolutely stunned.

I started to work on the little boy that I may have just killed. I couldn't think. I just worked on reflex. The local police arrived to help. Our dispatcher was notified that CPR was in progress, but she didn't know who was in cardiac arrest. That sent the other crews at our ambulance company into a frenzy.

Within ten minutes, there were two more ambulances on scene

to help with our rescue and life-saving efforts. With vigorous and aggressive advanced life support efforts, Bob and I were able to restore a pulse to the little boy. The other crews on scene quickly removed him and his father from the scene of the accident and sped off to the nearest hospital. Fortunately, the hospital was less than six miles away.

By that time, my boss was on the scene and took me to the same hospital as the two people whose lives I had forever changed. It was routine to have my blood sampled for any alcohol level or illicit drugs in situations like this. The blood turned out clean, but I sat there in a stunned state of consciousness. It all seemed so surreal. Did this all really happen or was I having a nightmare? Did I cause this? In my heart of hearts I didn't really know.

What I did know, was that I sure didn't get into this business to take lives or cause a loss of life. I wanted to be a part of the people who really did God's work of helping their fellow humans by easing pain and saving lives. I wanted to be counted with those who gave aid and comfort to people in their greatest time of need. As I sat in the emergency room watching the doctors and nurses struggle to stabilize the injuries sustained in the accident, I prayed for the man and child, and wished that fate hadn't brought us all together in one tragic instant of miscalculation or indecision.

In the blink of an eye, everything had changed. That family would never again be the same—and to a much lesser degree neither would mine. I wondered, *What do I do now? How in the hell did this happen? Who is going to figure this out? Why did this happen?* I wondered, *Was I at fault? Was the father laying unconscious on the hospital gurney, at fault? Were we both at fault? Do we both share the blame for this awful incident?*

If I were to blame, how would I ever live with the knowledge that I caused such a tragedy? If the father were to blame, how would he ever heal from the pain of knowing that he may have just killed his son? In the deepest part of my heart, I earnestly hoped that he just didn't see or hear me coming, and he wasn't trying to beat me to the intersection. If that were indeed the case, how on earth would he ever reconcile that with himself, his wife, or with God?

When a vehicle tries to beat an ambulance through an intersection, it does so when the driver attempts to quickly turn left at an intersection, rather than to move to the right, or just sit still. They attempt to continue on their way before the emergency vehicle approaches and passes through the traffic junction. Anyone who has ever driven a police car, fire truck, or ambulance, has seen this many times. In that situation, I was really praying that I too, was just in a bad place at a bad time, and that I wouldn't be found culpable in the accident.

As I sat there, so many things went through my mind. Most of them were just trying to replay in microseconds—the three or four seconds that encompassed the collision. I replayed that in my head for what seemed like hours. I began to think of what it was that got me into this business in the first place? Would I have been better off being a carpenter like my father, or a welder like my brother?

I thought that if I had been doing anything else, I wouldn't be here now. It was at that instant, I felt as guilty as hell. My head told me I did the right thing. But I think, because I wasn't hurt at all, and that the other two people were so badly hurt, that I must be at fault. If that were the case, how could I ever make things right again?

I knew I wouldn't be able to. You never can. At that moment I wished I were working on one of my grandparent's farms. I began to think back to a tougher, but simpler life when honest work didn't hurt anybody. When life was straightforward you always knew where you stood and what had to be done.

I grew up, and still reside, in southwest Michigan. Our town was so small that we only had a three-man police department, and the area had two small all-volunteer fire departments. One fire department was for the small township in which I lived, and one for the smaller city which the township surrounded on three sides. Lake Michigan bordered us on the west side.

In the summers there were constants that I could always count on. The first, was that my brother and I got butch haircuts from my mother. The second, was that there would always be a neighborhood softball game to get in on— if there weren't chores to do around the house, or on my paternal grandparent's farm across the street.

14

The farm had a little bit of everything, ponies, pigs, chickens, ducks, geese and an ornery billy goat that was more like a household pet. For a brief period of time Grandpa, would buy a beef cow to raise, then have it butchered to share the meat with my Dad, and my aunts and uncles. But that only happened three times, as Grandpa said he got too attached to the cows to have them slaughtered.

His farm had a wide variety of crops that usually consisted of corn or soybeans. I distinctly remember baling hay, picking potatoes, tomatoes, peppers, and strawberries. If that wasn't enough, my maternal grandparents were serious grape farmers. So a lot of the time, even if there was a softball game at the ready, my brother and I would be busy working in one of the several large vineyards that covered their many acres.

If one of the farms didn't require our labor, my mother made sure that at the least we were mowing or raking the big yard around our house, and doing the chores expected of us each day. Even though I didn't much care for it at the time, she was developing a strong work ethic and an inner toughness within my brother John and me that would serve us well in adult life.

In 1968, before my eleventh birthday, my mom's father died on St. Patrick's Day. After Grandpa's funeral I spent every weekend helping Grandma. In the summers I lived on the farm, and didn't return home again until it was time to go back to school in the fall. During those years I remember hearing the fire whistle going off five or six times a week. The respect, the danger, the sirens, and the inherent feeling of being really important, were thoughts that for me were irresistible.

The township fire department was just over a half mile from my home. That meant that the fire trucks would come blazing by with their lights flashing and sirens wailing. Man-o-man, that was some really cool stuff. As I entered high school, I remember wanting to become a Michigan State Trooper. I went to the high school library and logged onto a microfiche machine (computers weren't available to students in the early 70's) that had all of the information about being a state trooper. I found the physical requirements required a height taller than my five-feet-nine inches. But, that requirement was being lowered every so often, so I wasn't overly concerned about that. I was a high school athlete, and therefore knew the other physical attributes were not going to be any problem. I also didn't have problems with academic requirements.

Halfway through my junior year, I got back onto the microfiche just to make sure I was lined up academically for my senior year. I wanted to make sure that I hadn't left anything out that would benefit my chances to attain my goal of eventually becoming a state trooper. As I scrolled down, there it was, the dagger that figuratively stabbed me right through my heart. I needed to have a minimum of uncorrected 20/40 eyesight. I was nearly blind without corrective lenses. I was just devastated.

Consequently, I just floated through my senior year in high school without a plan. Watching television was a way I could get my mind off of my new reality, that apparently was not going to include a career in law enforcement. As it was every Saturday night I watched a patrol cop show *Adam-12,* and a new show called *EMERGENCY.* Of course, I always watched all of the cop shows such as the *FBI, Dragnet, Police Story, The Fugitive,* and even Angie Dickinson in *Police Woman.* Heck, I even watched the old Dick Tracy cartoons when I was real young.

In EMERGENCY, two firefighters had been cross-trained in emergency medicine and became paramedics. They were stationed with a crew of firefighters that ran an engine company. To me, those firemen were like emergency room doctors; they saved lives and were really impressive. What a great concept. At the time, I didn't even know whether or not it was conceptually real or a work of fiction. Did those firemen, called "paramedics," named Johnny Gage and Roy DeSoto, actually exist, or were they dreamed up like Luke Skywalker and Han Solo of *Star Wars'* fame?

It was a great show with great stories of these guys fighting big fires at oil refineries, saving heart attack victims, and rescuing kids who had drowned. I wanted to find out. I needed to find out. Within a few short weeks of watching Roy and Johnny perform life saving and life altering rescues, I was hooked. I knew the township and the city fire departments' personnel ran the all-volunteer ambulance service. So it was my goal to get on one of the fire department staffs.

Although my family lived in the township, Dad was the captain on the city fire department. My parents owned property in the city, which made him eligible to be a member of the city fire department. Years before, he knew the city fire chief and just asked if they needed help. The chief said yes. Since Dad was a self-employed carpenter and home builder, it was easy for him to respond to fire alarms. With his connections, he got me on the department in 1976, a month after I graduated from high school.

Back then, you didn't need all of the fire-fighting training you do today. You just learned as you went along. What I really wanted though, was to work on the ambulance. For that I needed to be certified in Advanced First Aid, which was offered through the American Red Cross. During my senior year in high school I did obtain CPR training through the American Heart Association. Just before graduation I took the CPR instructors training course. It was an all-day Saturday event at a local hospital that included doing one-man CPR for forty-five minutes nonstop. That afternoon, I became a certified American Heart Association CPR instructor.

At some point in the late summer of 1976, I learned of an Emergency Medical Technician (EMT) program at the community college that was to start in January 1977. The training was very formal and highly regimented. It had all kinds of medical jargon and terminology. It was where the people laying on the ambulance cots became "patients", not victims.

An old geezer named Lloyd, taught the class. He was tall, kind of hunched forward, and had incredibly thick bifocal glasses. I believe he was a retired high school teacher who had an acute interest in pre-hospital care for the sick and injured. Lloyd's enthusiasm for EMS allowed him to teach again—albeit on a part time basis. He not only taught for the local community college, but he also taught First-Aid, Advanced First-Aid, and many CPR classes for the local Red Cross.

He shared with us how he was constantly going to city and township meetings all over our county to strongly advocate the need for better-trained EMS personnel. He also visited several of the area police and fire departments to urge them to upgrade their first-aid training. He was passionate about the need for improved

EMS, and tireless in his promotion of this all-important cause. He was truly an example of what one man can accomplish if he has an unwavering devotion and a laser-like focus on an objective.

On the first day of the EMT class, I was issued a book that was about three inches thick, weighed about three pounds and included a workbook and several folders. The class met from 6-9 p.m. Monday and Thursday evenings for about five months. During this time, I was working eight hours a day for my aunt and uncle who owned a plastic injection mold factory. The factory was clean enough to eat off the floor and my aunt and uncle really bent over backwards to make me happy. Thirty years later, I'm still grateful for the patience and love they showed me. But the industrial and manufacturing industry just wasn't for me.

At that time the State of Michigan had no formal licensure for EMT's. If you passed, you were issued a certificate of successful completion from the college, and then you could apply for an ambulance attendant's license. By today's standards, it was really archaic. But that's how it was.

While I was a month or so away from completing my EMT training, I had heard that the township board of trustees were looking to hire someone full time because the all-volunteer service was having trouble staffing people during the day. Almost all of the guys on the two fire departments had full-time jobs during the day. So, after I completed the training, I made my sales pitch and was hired. That also meant I had to quit the city fire department and become a volunteer for the township fire department.

I officially started my new duties June 1, 1977, for the tidy sum of $8,500 dollars a year. My work schedule was from 8 a.m. to 5 p.m. Monday through Friday. If I happened to run on an ambulance call outside of those hours, I was paid like each of the firemen, $15 per call. Early on and during the course of my career, I experienced things that would make many people quit and just go back to a simple life with simple means —no lives to save or lose. That car accident with the young boy and his father didn't end after the boy died.

My boss Bill, at Medic 1, called me at my home to inform me of the boy's death before it got into the newspapers. I very much appreciated that, but the news hit me like a sledgehammer. At that instant, I wished that I had done anything, including rolling the ambulance over, in order to avoid hitting that little car. As I understand it, there were elements in the community that pressured the police department to bring a criminal charge.

One of the local churches (during a regular Sunday service) somehow or another brought up the accident, and basically bad-mouthed that "evil ambulance driver" for killing the little boy and injuring his father. The only reason I know any of this was because a retired truck driver, who saw the whole accident and testified at the pre-trial on my behalf, was sitting in that church on that same Sunday. He told my Medic-sponsored lawyer the distasteful details of the pastoral smear job.

I was charged with negligent homicide. I was stunned at the severity of the charge and really pissed off in being charged with anything at all. At the same time, I was scared about the real possibility of a prison sentence and being separated from my wife, and at the time our two small children. Even with a best-case scenario following a felony conviction (and perhaps lucky enough to avoid criminal confinement), my paramedic license would have been gone forever, and my career in EMS would end.

With local, small town politics as they usually are—and people only hearing one side of the story—I guess I shouldn't have been surprised. The county sheriff's department called Medic 1 and told my boss that I was to surrender myself. So, the next day I came in all dressed in my three-piece suit, and looked to get things straightened out. That didn't happen.

Instead, my boss and I were immediately escorted downstairs. Once there, I remember having to remove my shoes, the belt from my pants, my necktie, and everything in my pants pockets. I was then marched in front of a camera to have my mug shot taken. I don't know if I ever felt so low and so humiliated. I refused to look into the camera, mostly because I didn't know what else I could do to protest this whole ordeal. As the deputy explained the finger-printing procedure to me, he manually rolled each of my fingers through the ink pad, and transferred my fingerprints onto paper.

I began to feel more than just physically manipulated by an

unjust charge. I felt like a half-stripped common criminal. My thoughts were of a failed family man, and now a wasted life put on hold. I thought about all of the hard work that would be for naught. Mostly, I thought about the shame I brought to my family's good name.

By this time the anger and fury that was bottled up inside came spilling out. While I was being fingerprinted, I was really being obstinate and uncooperative. I know the deputies were only doing their jobs, but at the time I didn't care. After most of the finger printing was done, I had to put my four inked-stained fingers on a particular place on the paper alongside the other finger prints. Instead, I slammed my fingers across all of the other prints just to ruin the whole thing.

The deputy lost his cool as well and yelled, "Nice job asshole!"

With my boss standing right next to me, I just screamed back, "I don't give a shit!"

Bill immediately got into my ear and said in the sternest of voices, "Calm down, Jim! Calm down!"

I yelled back, "I can't calm down, goddamn it. This is such bullshit! I can't calm down!"

Finally, I calmed myself enough to finish the fingerprinting, and then I was released on my own recognizance. A week or two later it went to pre-trial, where the assistant district attorney and the local police chief (in whose jurisdiction the accident happened) battled my lawyer for more than two hours. But, the judge threw out the case and dismissed all of the charges.

Among other things, the judge stated that I, as an emergency driver of an ambulance, "...had a right to expect that other drivers on the road would do the right thing." I remember the assistant district attorney was so upset that he just sat behind his desk on his side of the courtroom, and was just as red-faced as he could be. My attorney smiled as the judge read the law and how it applied to me and my particular circumstances. He in fact, had supplied the judge with what he was now reading as part of his findings for no-cause in my prosecution.

Several weeks later the civil suit was filed. At the time I didn't know anything about this type of prosecution. I couldn't reconcile myself to the fact that now I was being sued for something I wasn't guilty of. It didn't make sense. When I complained about this type of legal action to my next lawyer, he said that the criminal complaint had nothing to do with the civil complaint. As it turned out, after several depositions, Medic 1 was the only entity that was held liable. After a couple of negotiations between the plaintiff's attorney and Medic's insurance company, the whole thing was settled out of court. The entire episode took more than a year.

Probably the worse for me was how I felt from my continuous reflection of the collision, and the feelings of doubt and guilt. Not guilt from doing something wrong, but guilt of not doing something different. But what? Although my wife, relatives, and many of our friends were publicly and privately very supportive of my plight, their words of encouragement held very little solace.

For a long time I seemed unable to focus on tasks at hand. I was easily agitated, and just felt a lot of self-doubt and a lacked sense of self worth. I remember it as being a terrible time for me as well as my family. Although I couldn't hardly imagine, I'm sure it was doubly awful for the family that lost their little boy that early morning.

***

The very first ambulance call I responded to was for a drug overdose. The patient was a female around twenty years old, who was essentially unconscious. She was lying in a mud puddle across the street from the entrance of Warren Dunes State Park (a Michigan State Park located at the southern tip of our township). The park is 650 acres of sunny beach and towering sand dunes, which makes it a summer weekend retreat for the Chicago crowd.

Even though I had all of this "book training," it was no substitute for practical, real, hands-on experience. After the two firemen made sure she was breathing, it was strictly a, Throw-her-on-the-cot-and-let's-go type of encounter. There was no checking of vital signs, no oxygen given, no physical or cognitive assessment at all. I thought, Yikes! Is this the only thing these guys do?

After my first twenty-five calls, I became comfortable and confident in what I was doing at the basic level. Looking back, I think how ignorant I was. Could you imagine thinking you knew what you were doing after running just a couple of dozen ambulance calls? The fact of the matter was, I just happened to have more formal training than the next guy.

As I started doing patient assessments—recording vital signs along with performing newer splinting techniques and all of the other things I was taught—it really irritated most of the firemen. They basically thought that transportation was the main treatment and that medical histories, assessments, and vital signs were just a big waste of time. I thought of the ambulance as just another tool to be used in caring for someone, just like a splint, the administration of oxygen, or how a bandage would be used.

Most of the guys on the fire department were between the ages of 40 and 60. I was just 19 years old. To me, they were basically a bunch of guys that belonged to a club more than operating a fire department. I'm sure to them I was a smart-assed kid who thought he knew it all. On top of that, I'm sure they were thinking, "We're not listening to the direction or even the ideas of any kid. After all, there isn't anything overtly wrong with the way things are going, so he can just kiss our asses."

Although he didn't have the power to impose any discipline on me, the volunteer fire chief was my immediate supervisor, and the rest of the department elected him. Consequently, I was going to have a tough time trying to change anything, so I put up with the basic unprofessionalism, indifference, and occasional fireman who had been drinking and (rarely) outwardly intoxicated.

In the mid-fall of 1977, I found out that the local doctors were going to put on an advanced EMT (better known as a paramedic) program. It was to be headed by a doctor originally from Tennessee named Dr. Robert Small, who had served in Vietnam in a M.A.S.H. unit as an anesthesiologist. One of the prerequisites was to have at least one year of experience as a basic EMT. I had only been a basic EMT for maybe five months. I talked with Dr. Small and lamented about the fact that I had not yet been an EMT a full year. I basically whined about the time line invoked, and I made it painfully obvious that I really wanted to get into this first-ever paramedic class. He simply said, "I'll see what I can do."

I got busy writing my letter of application, and spoke of my vision of EMS, and basically begged for one of the twenty-four spots in the class. I talked with our local doctor (who was my mother's cousin) for a letter of recommendation. He was happy to do so. I asked and got letters of recommendation from the township fire chief, the township supervisor, and clerk. I submitted them all to the local college where I previously had received my basic EMT training, and kept my fingers crossed.

They told me they would call if I were selected. After about two weeks I couldn't stand not knowing, so I called the college contact person. She said they had just finalized the list and I was number eight on that list. To say I was elated would be a huge understatement. I was literally jumping up and down in my office at the fire department.

At the same time, I was still having huge problems with a large number of the guys I worked with on the ambulance. Although some of them were really trying to do the right thing, the vast majority didn't give a damn about much of anything when it came to working on the ambulance. I really believe it was just a money issue for them.

In the meantime, I had gotten about six guys into an EMT class at the high school, where I taught the extrication part of the training. Extricating (or removing) someone out of a wrecked automobile, a train, or downed plane, is really something of an art form. It's a whole lot of fun to practice and extremely beneficial in times of need. Until those chosen few completed their training I was going to have to tolerate the firemen and their antics.

After the completion of the EMT program, I started to work with some of the new EMT's on ambulance calls. I did this by calling one of the new EMT's after the county would dispatch our ambulance. Until the late 1970's we didn't use pagers or walkie-talkie's, we used what we called "fire phones". You could tell the difference between a normal, everyday phone call as opposed to an emergency call by the ring of the phone. For an emergency call, the ring would be constant and uninterrupted.

The emergency number (also before 911) would ring in twenty different homes. Usually one of the first two or three guys to pick up the phone would answer the caller by saying: "Fire department," and then everyone else would listen in on the ensuing conversation. Typically, it would be either a private citizen or the county sheriff dispatch center calling to tell all of us if the emergency was medically related, or whether there was a fire. Sometimes the ambulance and the fire trucks were needed.

So what I did after answering the phone, when the need was just for the ambulance, was to say, "I have it handled." Then I would immediately call one of "my guys" and tell them we had an ambulance call. Since there were at times perhaps eight to ten times as many ambulance calls as there were fire calls in a given month, it wasn't long before the malcontents caught on to my end run around the rules.

By that time, there were vague physical threats aimed my way, which were little more than a bunch of guys just being ignorant, and basically spouting off and blowing off steam. But that all came to a head during a snowstorm late one night. The fire phone rang and I asked whether anyone wanted to run this particular call with me? For whatever reason, I didn't have one of the EMT's scheduled on duty. One firefighter, "Frank", said he would meet me at the station. I could tell by his slurred speech that he had been drinking.

I arrived at the fire station first—mostly because I only lived about a half mile away. When he arrived and climbed into the ambulance I could really smell the booze. So right off the bat, I was upset. During the early years of my tenure with EMS, there wasn't nearly the emphasis on sobriety in driving any kind of vehicle as there is today.

During this storm, a car had become stalled or disabled in the middle of a country road. There was at least two feet of snow around the car and more coming down. It looked like it had been there for quite a while. Then out of the dark, and through a heavy snowfall, came four snowmobiles. Three of the riders got past the car. However, the fourth one ran right into the back end of the car. I don't recall how fast he said he was moving, but it was fast enough to break one of his femurs.

When we rolled onto the scene our patient was lying in the snow complaining of pain to his left thigh. He had a heavy one-piece snowmobile suit on along with a full-faced helmet. He was conscious, alert, fully oriented, and had no other observable injuries. Since my fire-fighting companion was of little help, I enlisted the assistance of the other three riders to help put their buddy onto a backboard. His thigh literally looked as though he had an extra knee joint. I told him that his quadriceps muscles were in spasm, and until we got those muscles stretched out the pain was going to continue.

We picked up the backboard, gently set it on the ambulance cot, and loaded in the victim. I then retrieved a special splint called a HARE traction splint, which works great when applied properly.

Generally, it takes two people to apply the splint. One person needs to pull traction on the thigh (by pulling on the ankle) in the attempt to pull the spasm out of the quadriceps muscles, and to keep the broken ends of the bones apart. The other person is to apply the splint from the hip to past the end of the foot. But because my partner couldn't help, I had to do it myself. It is very difficult, but it is possible.

When I finished a head-to-toe assessment, I got busy applying this traction splint. Halfway through the one-person lengthy procedure, my partner opened one of the back doors to the ambulance and asked in a disgusted voice, "Are ya' ready to go yet, or not?"

I responded in a very terse voice, "No!" He then slammed the door shut, clearly irritated.

Here I am, wishing I could grow an extra hand to get this splint on my patient, and my partner was mad at me for not getting it done fast enough. What a surprise. As I finished and my patient's leg was feeling much better, I suddenly heard a bunch of laughter. One of the snowmobile riders yelled, "I'm sure glad I'm not having a heart attack!" I briskly walked around to the side of the ambulance to where the laughter was coming from.

As I turned the corner, I saw my partner urinating on the side of the ambulance. I was just aghast and totally embarrassed. I was embarrassed for me, my knuckleheaded partner, and the whole fire department. I mean, the name of the township was right there on the ambulance. What I saw said it all. To top it all off, he drove me—along with the patient—to the local hospital. Fortunately, we didn't run into a ditch or force a car off the road during our trek to the hospital in the snowstorm. We arrived at the emergency room without incident. In retrospect, I should have called for additional help before I even started to put on the traction splint, and my partner should have been relieved of duty right then and there. Then, I should have left his drunken ass sitting in the snow, waiting to talk with a police officer.

Tell me, did Roy and Johnny ever have to put up with that?

Chapter 2
THIS IS FOR REAL

As time went on, I needed clarification as to what my role was in the ambulance department. I talked to the township supervisor and wanted my position clarified as to whom exactly was running the ambulance-side of our emergency services. Is it going to remain with the fire chief, or since things were changing, is it going to be with me? I really needed to know.

The fire chief was really a good guy, but didn't know much about health or human sciences. Why would he? He was a full-time dairy farmer who probably heard as many complaints about me from some of the firemen as the complaints I made about some of them. Again, the majority of the firemen were great guys that didn't have any desire or wish to respond to or run ambulance calls. Besides a few incidents where they were unfair to others, I harbored no malice toward any of them whatsoever.

So, when I pressed the township supervisor about who was calling the shots, I reminded him that soon the State of Michigan would require at least one EMT on the ambulance during each call. And there wasn't a single fireman interested in any EMT training. Furthermore, when I told him what Frank had done at the scene of the snowmobile accident he couldn't believe it. He was so upset that he couldn't talk. After he regained his composure, he shook his finger at me and said, "Listen, you run this ambulance service like you think it should be run! From now on, you answer to me!"

That was all I needed to hear. I had been employed for approximately eighteen months, and I got busy directing the movement from fire phones, to a pager system that was in operation widely throughout the county. It was used to dispatch the many volunteer fire and ambulance services. The two local fire departments, as well as the ambulance service, were behind the times and the last to go to county dispatch. After we did that the die was cast. I immediately wrote a letter to the fire chief and in essence told him I was terminating the members of the fire department who ran ambulance calls.

The six or eight guys that had taken their EMT training and were interested in this type of public service, would now handle all ambulance calls. For me, it worked out just great. It probably goes without saying that there were plenty of pissed-off people. As a purely punitive measure, the firemen stated, since I was obviously more interested in running ambulance calls than running fire calls, I no longer needed to be a member of the fire department. So right in front of me during a regular fire meeting, they voted to kick me off the fire department. Of course there was no valid reason and absolutely no just cause. After all, I hadn't embarrassed an entire township by urinating on their fire truck.

Frank on the other hand, was never reprimanded for his classless actions. He stayed on the department for several more years and left on his own accord. For better or for worse, the ambulance and fire department operations were permanently separated. Like an ill-suited marriage, all parties were probably better off. The group of guys who received their EMT training were really a great bunch. I think of them every once and again from a distance of more than thirty-five years. I still have tremendous respect for all of them. For many years, they admirably served their community with professional and ethical distinction.

Since the ambulance service was now a separate organization, I got busy and wrote a rudimentary constitution, and a set of by-laws. Then during a couple of our meetings, we as a group, fine tuned it and made it permanent. It was a collective effort and something everybody could live with. We held two meetings a month. One was basically a business meeting, and the other was a training meeting where we would select a couple of pieces of equipment and practice their use. We would trade off being the patient or the rescuer, and then work at it until we were comfortable doing the exercise. We even got an old car and practiced extricating each other from it. It was really a fun time and an extraordinarily valuable learning experience.

***

You know how it is when things are going too well? Watch out, because something is going to smack you right in the chops. Officials from a small community and adjoining township wanted to know if it was possible to merge with our ambulance service? They were having problems staffing their ambulance during the day. I didn't see why it would be a problem, as we only ran on average of two calls per day, and they were running less than one per day. I really didn't think that running three calls per day rather than two was any big deal. After the small village and their surrounding township worked out the details and the money issues with our township, we annexed their service area into our own.

Now, I have to say that our township supervisor (and my boss) had been the supervisor for about thirty years. He ran everything. If he didn't want something to happen, it wouldn't. We did have a need for another ambulance. After all when it comes to EMS, if you are going to assume the duties and responsibilities of other areas, you had better be ready with enough staff as well as equipment. The ambulance service members looked at different makes and models, and we knew what was needed and wanted. However, the supervisor made it clear he was going to be the one to pick out the next ambulance.

Furthermore, it was going to be done with little to no input from the guys that would be responding with it, and working out of it. Like the fire chief, he too was a dairy farmer, but that was where the similarities ended. The supervisor had no clue what was needed; he just had to have the final say on each and every issue. What he picked out "for us" was a big, poorly constructed box unit, that rattled so loudly in the patient compartment that you could hardly be heard without yelling. As a result, it wasn't long before things were starting to go south with him.

I had just started my paramedic training. I distinctly remember spouting off that I was going to be some "big time paramedic" or some such thing. What a mistake that was. When Dr. Small talked with all of us on that first day and told us what we were in for, I thought, *What on God's green earth did I just sign up to do?* This was going to be nothing short of ten months of extremely intensive, in your face learning and training. It was also going to take about a thousand times as much studying as I ever did in high school. We were expected to maintain an 80% or above on each of our tests. If we fell below that for any length of time, we would be permanently excused from the class.

When I looked at the syllabus I just about passed out. This was going to be exponentially more labor intensive than the EMT course I had completed less than a year earlier. Plus, the practical hours involved were going to be significantly more. We spent at least 180 hours in the emergency rooms of two local hospitals. Considerable time was also spent in the intensive care and coronary care units, laboratory, and surgical departments—all of that, plus countless hours of studying.

The entire class was going to start with the first month being a whirlwind basic review of medical and traumatic emergencies, with an added advanced life support spin to each emergency. When we started the cardiology part of the class, which lasted four months, the cardiologist who was selected to teach it was a well-respected man by the name of Dr. Frank Bunker. As I recall, he had a very thick Spanish accent. You had to listen very carefully as not to miss what he was saying. I thought, *Gee-whiz, if this isn't hard enough, now I have to struggle through a language barrier too?*

He spoke for the first hour of each of the two-days-a-week classes. Then, an absolutely great woman by the name of Irma Hannah (the department head of emergency services at one of the local hospitals), took over for the remaining three hours. She was a nurse that really knew her stuff. For some reason she liked me and I thought the world of her. I often said, that if I had to have a second mom, it would have been Irma.

Reading EKG's is comparable to reading and interpreting hieroglyphics. For me it was really tough. I talked with Irma about it and she told me not to worry, and that it all would come together in an instant. Of course, she was right. It was like it all just snapped into place in a single day. In the meantime, the State of Michigan sent a list of objectives.

There were 103 written, and 105 practical objectives that needed to be mastered by the time each of us tested for our state licensure. Before the testing date, there was a massive amount of learning to do. With all of those objectives to cover, ten months isn't a long time. So the game plan was to listen intently, study your butt off, and then hopefully ask an intelligent question or two. After the cardiology part of the course was over we immediately started to go over all of the drugs that we would use; the vast majority was to treat cardiac dysrhythmias (abnormal heart rhythms).

There are more than two dozen dysrhythmias—more than half are considered problematic, and about six are deemed lethal. When we started to learn about the drugs and fluids that we would be using, there were more than twenty-five kinds, and each did something specific. We had to know the physiological effects of each drug—not to mention the correct dosage—routes of administration, indications, contraindications, and side effects. On top of that, some drugs have a synergistic effect when given together.

Obviously, there was a tremendous amount of information to learn to have a thorough understanding of all the medicines needed to administer to patients. When that part of the training was completed, you had to then combine it with the cardiology part, and then apply it to the appropriate patients. It was very complicated, and at times confusing.

What we were taught was drilled into us. Scenarios were given. Each time assessment, diagnosis, and treatment was closely critiqued. At each juncture your critical thinking and decisions are scrutinized. This is completely understandable when you realize that only on rare occasions would there be a doctor, nurse, or other medical professional at the scene of an emergency to assist. The problems encountered by all levels of EMS personnel vary widely. They range from maybe applying a bandage or something just as simple, to high-velocity trauma, gunshot wounds of all types, and cardiovascular emergencies—including cardiac arrest. In essence, you are on your own.

We were maybe two-thirds the way through the class when I received a written offer to work for an ambulance service that was municipally owned, called Medic 1. The service was centrally located in Benton Harbor, Michigan. At that time, they staffed three ambulances twenty-four hours a day, and served about 50,000 people in about ten communities.

Before and after I had received their offer, I had been asked several times by the guys that worked at Medic 1, if I wanted a job with them? They were probably twenty times busier than the small town and township I currently served, even with the acquisition of the even smaller township and village we had added. That was attractive to me. But, what I really wanted at the time was to be the king in my little kingdom.

While I thought so, I really wasn't the king. Paramedics operate under a medical doctor's license and we have a large and extensive set of protocols to guide us. That particular doctor is known as the Project Medical Director (PMD), and he is the king of the castle. Dr. Small was our first one. I told him of my ideas and he shot the notion of me having my own "kingdom" down right away. He said the best thing that could happen was if the communities I served would join the other communities that operated the Medic 1 Ambulance service.

Being young and dumb, I still thought I could run my own autonomous advanced life support ambulance. To do so, I was going to have to make a deal with Medic 1 ambulance and the hospital-based medical control. So the proposition was, that I would take some of the area that Medic served, that bordered the north side of my township. At that time, Medic was having a difficult time covering that small area in a timely fashion. That would add about ten square miles to my coverage area. With that, I thought I could operate my own advanced life support (ALS) service. Once again, I was incredibly naïve.

During this time I got the go-ahead to purchase a couple of relatively specialized pieces of equipment. The first piece was something that looked like the cot part of an ambulance stretcher. It was a machine that did CPR for you. It worked great when you had to carry someone in cardiac arrest, down a flight of stairs, or something similar to that.

The other, was something called an "Amb-pack." It actually was is a cardiac monitor and defibrillator wrapped in a hard metal shell, that could take getting dropped or kicked around in due course of an emergency response. Now we had the capability to monitor the patient's heart rhythm, or defibrillate (shock) that same patient's heart, if necessary. We were clearly moving toward a high-technology type of pre-hospital medical care.

By this time I was finishing up my training, and was rated as either second or third in the class (depending on the latest test score). Of the twenty-four people that started the class, only twelve finished. Of those, only five received a license. It was a long, tough, and grueling ordeal. If you really didn't want it, there was no way you would ever get through it.

Upon successfully completing the paramedic course, the five of us had to wait about a month for a test date. I spent that time going over and over all of the piles of information I had accumulated over the previous ten months. I learned we would take our test in Lansing at the Michigan Department of Public Health (MDPH). The group of us piled into one car and traveled to the state's capitol. Once there, we endured five solid hours of written testing. You had to pass each of the tests with at least 80%, or you would have to do it all again. As a great amount of preparation and a little bit of luck would have it, all of us passed on our first attempt.

After our successful completion of those three tests, we were invited back to take a practical examination. That was almost an all-day event. We thought that the practical portion would be easy—or at least easier than the written part. We were in for yet another surprise. The officials at the state that administered the test had several "stations" set up for us. They would be used to test and evaluate our skills we had learned over the past months, as well as our acquired level of expertise. I don't recall all of them now, but I remember a "mega-code" station where you had to run a cardiac arrest from the moment you happened upon a "victim", to when you delivered a "patient" to the emergency department.

There were several different scenarios that tossed about every arrhythmia possible. You had to tell the tester or evaluator everything. Nothing was left to chance. That meant CPR, intubation, checking lung sounds, evaluating effective CPR, placement of chest leads, administration of oxygen, and all of the pharmacological interventions, and on and on. If you didn't do it right, exactly right, it was "see you another day".

I remember the intubation stations, IV stations, cardiac rhythm recognition stations, and situation stations. The "situation station" was similar to the mega-code station. It had a more wide range of scenarios that they tested and evaluated you on than the mega-code station. One situation might be: Someone was unconscious and bleeding out of both ears after their car struck a tree. Another might be: An eight-year-old child had just been pulled from the bottom of a pool and didn't have a pulse. Another might be: A known drug addict is found disoriented or combative. There were dozens of scenarios, and they all were different in content as well as in their scope of treatment.

That station was pressure-packed and intense. To make things just a little more arduous, the examiner had a stopwatch that ticked so loudly, it added to the distraction. You had three minutes to do a complete assessment and decide on your treatments—both on a basic and an advanced life-support level—and get your patient into the ambulance. So here I am, trying to think through all of this while this "gong" is ticking away.

I saw my buddy Mark Parren, who looked as though he had been through a wrestling match. He looked disheveled and was sweating up a storm. I remember saying, "Sweating a little bit there, Parren?"

Without missing a beat, he snapped back saying, "No worse than you!" He was right. I hadn't really noticed, but I was also showing signs of stress. My hands were cold; I too was sweating profusely, not to mention just being really on edge. After all, just one slip-up and it could be over for the day. I knew there wasn't any chance that any one of us, after coming so far, wanted to fail.

To go home, knowing you would have to return to test again, was worse than any other possibility. Thinking back, I thought there was a little luck involved in whether you passed or failed, but very little. You either knew what you were doing or you didn't. Considering the awesome and many responsibilities paramedics have, it shouldn't be easy. The tax-paying public deserved that much.

We all passed! I remember feeling like I just ran through a hail of arrows, and had slain a dragon. I was contemplating all of the hard work, the unending studying, the countless clinical hours, and just couldn't believe I made it through along with four of my buddies from the class. We knew if we got through all of that, it was time for a wild unbridled celebration. On the way home on that warm October day, we had the windows open and were whooping and hollering and having a good 'ole time.

We stopped in Kalamazoo at a restaurant and bar called Bilbo's where we ate, and gave toasts to Dr. Small, Irma Hannah, and Dr. Bunker. They were the pillars of the program and were largely responsible for our successful completion through this first-ever paramedic program. Most of the advanced life-support measures that we enjoy today are directly attributable to their good work, dedication, and vision. Many hundreds of lives have been saved and the morbidity of perhaps thousands has been minimized due to their dedicated teaching and tireless instruction.

After I arrived home, my parents met me anxiously at the door.

"Well?" Mom said nervously.

"Come over here and give a paramedic a big hug," I said, with a wide grin.

They knew how hard the classes and everything had been. Mom even shed a tear or two. A week later I received an application for licensure as an Advanced Emergency Medical Technician. The license fee was only three dollars. Mom threw me a big celebration party where relatives, friends, EMT's, the fire chief, and the township clerk all attended.

In late November of 1978, I received my first paramedic license. During the next eight months things proceeded along with my attempts to secure an Advanced Life Support (ALS) ambulance. The whole ALS thing was going to be controlled from a medical aspect and not a geopolitical position. That meant Dr. Small would act as the PMD and would ultimately be in charge of all EMS services in the county. It also meant that the power-obsessed supervisor from our township would have no control of the actual operation of the ambulance. The communities may in fact own the ambulance and the contents and equipment, but who would work, how they would work, and so forth, would be an issue for the PMD.

Enter our township supervisor. While I was delivering a patient to the local hospital, Dr. Small happened to be on duty. He approached me and said, "I have to talk to you before you leave the hospital."

I'm thinking, *Well that's never good news.* After I had finished giving the patient report to the attending nurse, I helped get the ambulance back in order and did my own paperwork on the call I had just completed. When I finished, I lightly tapped on the doctors' lounge door and stepped inside to see him sitting in his recliner.

"What's up?" I said.

"I understand you won't be getting ALS," he said with a bit of anger in his voice.

Being somewhat shocked and incredulous at his off-handed statement I said, "What do you mean, we won't be getting any ALS?"

He gets up out of his chair, looks me right in the eye, and without so much as a blink, says with a little more anger in his voice, "I just talked with your supervisor yesterday and he said you guys don't need Advanced Life Support."

I couldn't believe it. I snapped back, "Listen, we need it a whole lot more than around here. You're only three minutes from this hospital. Christ all mighty, we have to travel thirty minutes to get here!"

He shrugged his shoulders and said, "Well, if I know your supervisor, you guys aren't going to get it."

I felt like somebody just kicked me in the groin. When I left the hospital I was stunned, emotionally hurt, and as angry as I had been in a long time. As my partner that day was driving us back to the station, I didn't say much at all. My mind was whirling. I knew immediately what had happened. Since the township supervisor could not control the new and burgeoning service, he didn't want it.

Politically, it was the most self-serving thing I've ever witnessed on a local level. It had so many negative implications. The idea of power meant everything. The notion of how many people could benefit from this type of ambulance service meant nothing to him.

At first, I thought the hard work that I had done to promote our service, and to help improve and enhance our emergency care, was wasted. But I was wrong. Progress can be slowed, but it is never stifled——at least not for very long. Soon there were going to be mandates from the state that would dictate that even Basic Life Support Service ambulances would be under the direct operational authority of medical control. It was just at the time, I thought that an opportunity to help the citizens in our service area had been missed.

I knew now that I would leave the township ambulance service. From a professional point of view I couldn't stay, even if I had wanted. If I couldn't practice pre-hospital medicine at my present place of employment, I would have to go somewhere else. It was just the blatant selfishness that I found so incredible and despicable. When I got back to the station, I immediately wrote a letter of resignation and took it over to the township clerk's house. I informed her what had transpired and how betrayed I felt. She had a sympathetic ear, but that was about as far as it would go. My letter informed her that I would finish out the week. I took off the rest of the day. That was in the middle of July, 1979.

The next day, I picked up the phone and called Medic 1 Ambulance and talked with a guy by the name of Jeff Kimber. He had just been named interim director of that service and was one of the many guys who were always after me to jump ship, and join Medic.

"Hey Kimber, this is Jim Stine and I'm looking for a job."

Jeff shot back, "Are you serious?"

Half laughing I yelled back, "Hell yes, I'm serious! I just quit the township!"

"When do you want to start?"

I thought about it for a moment and figured I needed a couple of weeks off to decompress, and declared, "How about the first of August?"

"Sounds great. Be here at 8 a.m.

***

When I first arrived, I was warmly welcomed by a bunch of guys that I had gotten to know over the last two years. They didn't make much money, but with their level of dedication, it was plain to see that they had EMS in their blood. At that time, Medic 1 had three ambulances that were on duty twenty-four hours a day. Two months before, Medic purchased an ambulance that would be outfitted and stocked with the equipment specifically used by just paramedics. Up to that point in time, Medic was just a basic life support (BLS) service, like every other ambulance in the county.

Of the five students who tested and passed almost ten months before, three of us were now employed by Medic 1. Two other guys from out of town were already employed at Medic 1 before I arrived. They were also inexperienced paramedics, waiting before the three of us got licensed, to work on the first ever ALS unit within our county.

Medic worked closely with the two local hospitals on issues of medical control, pharmaceuticals (including narcotics security), medical protocols that would be used by the five paramedics, and how we would interface with the emergency room staff. Finally, we obtained the needed and specialized equipment that was required by the State of Michigan to become licensed, and to operate as an advanced life-support ambulance.

To fill out our two-man teams for the three shifts, Medic needed a sixth paramedic, which they didn't have. However, the company wasn't going to wait an unnecessary second in putting the ALS ambulance on the road and into action. After all, it had been nearly ten months since we had become paramedics, and even though we continued with little study sessions, our practical skills were deteriorating. We were starting to forget the special technique used in intubation and the delicate touch for IV cannulation. That was really bad.

We were caught in a quandary. When we were students, we could work in the emergency room and put into practice all of the skills we had learned. However, the hospital's insurance carrier apparently conveyed to the administration that since we were no longer students, we would not be covered under their malpractice insurance plan.

When it was time to put the paramedics together into teams of two, Dr. Small made the decision to put Mark Parren and Mark Philotoff together as one team. Parren and Philotoff were two of the guys who became licensed with me. Greg Holda and Greg Pruitt were the second team. That left one shift to cover.

To make the needed third crew, I was selected to work with a basic EMT. That meant I had to do all of the advanced procedures. The advanced airway management, IV cannulation, drug therapy, EKG interpretation, and defibrillation would be solely my responsibility. I was excited at the opportunity and I looked forward to the pressure of being the only paramedic on-duty within a forty-mile radius.

At the same time I had the feeling of trepidation over the thought of something going terribly wrong. The reason I was chosen to work with a basic guy wasn't because I was better than anyone else, far from it. It was because I had the most clinical experiences. So, Dr. Small wanted one of the better EMT's to work with me. Jeff Kimber, our interim manager at Medic, chose a fellow by the name of Dave Hawkins. Dave knew the service area like the back of his hand and was comfortable in the back end of an ambulance too. He perhaps wasn't the best, but he was certainly one of the top EMT's working at Medic.

When we started there was much trial and error. My partner, Dave did all he could do to take the pressure off of me. He did all of the basic life support (BLS) procedures, as there are always many things to do. On or around the first of September 1979, the new ALS ambulance went into operation. Dave Hawkins and I were the first crew to operate in it that first day. To say that I was just a little tense at the idea of being the only paramedic on duty that first day, would be a huge understatement. At that time we knew we were in a unique situation, but neither of us had any idea how effective we would ultimately be. Luckily, we would not have to wait long to find out our worth.

At age 21, I was at the scene of a cardiac arrest. Did I really know what to do, now that it was live and in color? Would I do the right things in the right order? In the middle of my pressure-packed moment of doubt, I stopped for a second and thought to myself, *Hey doofus, it's not about you! It's about this patient and his life being in your hands. So get it right, the first time!*

Before the advent and realization of pre-hospital Advanced

Cardiac Life Support (ACLS), the only treatment an EMS provider would be able and authorized to do in regards to a victim of cardiac arrest is to start CPR, put in an oral airway, and ventilate the patient with a bag-valve-mask (BVM) device. Then your patient was quickly placed on the ambulance cot and was whisked off to the closest hospital.

Now, with advanced training and high-tech diagnostic equipment everything was different. It would forever be different. Instead of utilizing an oral airway, it was now possible to secure an airway through an advanced procedure called intubation. That means a hollow, semi-rigid plastic tube is introduced into the oral airway, and placed inside the trachea (a.k.a. windpipe), with the end of it attached to the BVM which was fastened to an oxygen bottle.

With just that much being accomplished, you have done several extremely valuable things for your patient. First and foremost, you've protected the airway from foreign matter (usually vomit) getting into the lungs. Also, keeping air out of the stomach is hugely beneficial as well. Without a doubt, the biggest benefit is that you can deliver as much as 100% of oxygen to a very secure airway. During the early moments of the cardiac arrest, I opened the airway box, selected the size of the tube needed, grabbed my laryngoscope, and within a few short seconds had successfully intubated the patient. So far, so good.

As the EMT's performed CPR, I started the IV and initiated drug therapy. Dave attached the chest leads from our heart monitor so I was able to see the rhythm our patient's heart was exhibiting.

With all of the new and advanced procedures to do, the four of us were really busy. About ten minutes into this ordeal, Medics' third ambulance arrived on the scene. It wasn't because we necessarily needed them; it was because I think the two guys in that ambulance wanted to say that they also got in on the very first ALS call in the county. As luck would have it, we defibrillated the patient three or four times before his heart started beating. He had a good blood pressure and now was ready to be taken to Mercy Hospital in Benton Harbor.

With all of our basic and advanced life support efforts we were probably on the scene a minimum of twenty-five minutes. This was a far cry from the quick "throw and go" routine we used to do for cardiac arrest patients by just getting them to the hospital, and not working on them on the scene. It was, and remains a quantum leap forward in patient care for the most seriously ill or injured people that need EMS.

Although I called Mercy prior to our arrival there, the staff on duty that day were stunned to see this guy hooked up and attached to the IV's, and the cardiac monitor (not to mention being intubated) as we came rushing through the doors. They were astounded to see that we had done essentially everything that is initially done by them in the first thirty minutes of a patient's arrival to any emergency room. Some of them didn't have any idea we had this type of capability.

As the six of us contemplated what we had just done and had been a part of, there were no shortages of high five's and back slapping hugs. Our first advanced life-support call was a memorable success for us. We learned that the patient (who had went into cardiac arrest due to a stroke) had died the next day.

After that particular call, everything went to hell in a hand basket. There are many skills that paramedics have to master. Patient assessment, EKG interpretation, and diagnosing, are at the top of the list. However, there are mainly only two physical skills that paramedics really do on a regular basis. The most prevalent one is starting IV's. The second skill is endotracheal intubation; the act of placing a hollow tube into your patient's trachea (wind pipe) to either breathe for them or assist in their inadequate breathing. If your particular patient needs to be intubated and you are for whatever reason unable to successfully do so, you may very likely deliver a corpse to your local emergency room.

For about two months after what was a first successful call, it seemed as though I couldn't do those two physical skills properly. In regards to the people who were now my patients that presented with severely compromised airways, I couldn't seem to place the tube properly. For those who found themselves lying on my ambulance cot in need of an IV, I kept on missing or rupturing their veins. It was as though my whole technique on these vitally important skills eluded me for some unknown reason.

The impact of those two months was brutal on me. Much worse than that, the impact on some of my patients may have been fatal. I'm not being overly dramatic, I was the only paramedic on duty within at least fifty miles. If the patient really needed a paramedic— for better or for worse, I was it!

During the building of a shopping mall in Benton Harbor, a heavy equipment operator collapsed. When I arrived, he was in cardiac arrest. I tried to intubate him, but missed on several attempts. My partner Dave ventilated him by using the BVM. Of course the patient vomited from the air that went into the stomach, and then aspirated the vomit into his lungs. Once that happens, the patient is in real trouble.

Even though we were able to place an IV in the patient's arm and start drug therapy, he never responded, and his color never improved from the dark blue in which we found him. It all stemmed from his severely compromised airway. I learned then and there, if you don't have an airway, you don't have a viable patient. More than thirty years later, I still believe that completely.

As I recall, that particular patient was probably in his mid 40s. He very well may have had a wife and kids at home that depended on his love and support each and every day. Here I was, charged with doing what is medically necessary and within the realm of my paramedic training and responsibility to save his life. I felt I was failing miserably. I had seriously thought of quitting the business altogether. I may not have been costing people their lives, but I was doing precious little to keep the grim reaper at bay.

The first rule of any kind of medicine is "do no harm." I was harming plenty of people, literally, on a daily basis. I just couldn't understand it. It got to the point that I was really dreading going into work. I had shot my big mouth off many months ago that I was going to be this big-time paramedic and save the planet. But, up to this point and time I was just a big flop. As it were, if one of the other paramedics from a different shift was having a bad day, they at least had their paramedic partner there to start the IV or intubate their patient, or whatever advanced skill that needed to be done. But not me. For better or for worse, I was all there was. Lately it had been for the worse.

My failings didn't go unnoticed. Dr. Small was keeping an extremely watchful eye on all of the new paramedics in this new system of delivering pre-hospital medical care.

"Jim, you're all that we have," Dr. Small said in stern disappointment. "Your technique is failing you for some reason and you have got to get it straightened out. The reason I selected you in the first place to be the paramedic to work with a basic (EMT) was because you had the best clinical experience. I know you can do it, so do it!"

By now I was depressed. I had no confidence and was as mad as hell. To top it all off, the pressure of being the only paramedic on duty was now accented by Dr. Small throwing the gauntlet down of getting my act together. Mostly though, I felt really bad for all of the patients and their families that I may have let down.

One day while at the hospital, a car came screeching up to the emergency room entrance, the horn was frantically honking. My partner Dave and I, along with a couple of the emergency room nurses, went out to see a woman who said her husband was complaining of chest pain. She ended up delivering a corpse. She said her husband had stopped talking to her about a mile or so into their twelve-mile trip. When we got him out of the car and onto a hospital gurney, he was cyanotic, his eyes were fixed, and dilated. The hospital staff was quick, aggressive, and efficient. They also were quite unsuccessful. He had been "not talking" too long.

After his widow finished her grieving, he was just laying on the emergency room bed waiting to be taken to the morgue. After resuscitation efforts are ceased, death has been declared, and family members have been given time to view and grieve the loss of their loved one, we may get to practice advanced airway management on the body. After the man's loved ones left the room, two of the finest nurses on duty at the time (Jan and Colleen) said, "Alright Jim, lets find out what you're not doing properly."

They watched me and analyzed my technique in intubation. They immediately saw my flaw and corrected it. It was just a little thing, but it apparently made all of the difference. In fact, after I had intubated him properly with the guidance of my two nurse friends, I removed the tube from the man's trachea, (extubated) and re-intubated him three additional times without a problem.

Next, they pulled me into the nurses' break room, and with a fist full of IV catheters in hand said, "Okay, let's find out what you're not doing right on these simple IV's you're not hitting."

Believe it or not—and much to my dismay—they both rolled up their sleeves and watched me poke holes into their arms. Again, my problem was the smallest of a technical error. It was easily corrected. I still lacked a whole lot of experience, but things went much, much better. Thanks to Jan and Colleen, my career got back on track again, and most importantly, my confidence flourished. I will never forget their kindness, concern, and their willingness to bleed on my behalf.

Chapter 3
VOLUNTEERS AND MFR'S

There is a huge group of people who have a positive impact on nearly everything paramedics and EMT's do on a daily basis. They are the civically-minded volunteers who offer their time as medical first responders. Typically in the medical setting, volunteers are those groups of people that respond from their everyday lives to come to the assistance of someone in need. Volunteers could be Medical First Responders (MFR's), Emergency Medical Technicians (EMT's), and sometimes—but not usually, paramedics.

They come from many backgrounds and walks of life to help their fellow citizen in a time of need. It may be volunteering to help out on a food drive or donating blood. It may be as profound as serving in the military or helping in a variety of ways in the wake of huge natural disasters. Usually their efforts go unheralded, unappreciated, and with little fanfare. To the ordinary person, they may seem at times invisible. To the professional paramedic and other emergency care providers, the MFR's place is essential in successful emergency health care.

Usually, paramedics with all of their essential equipment, advanced life support skills, and medicines are just too far away. So, an MFR may arrive first. Any paramedic worth his or her salt will tell you just how important quality medical first responder's can be. It can't be overstated.

Consider this: Someone has a witnessed sudden cardiac arrest and the local 911 system is activated. An advanced life support ambulance is dispatched but doesn't arrive for ten to twelve minutes. The person who called for emergency medical assistance doesn't know, or doesn't attempt CPR, and there are no Medical First responders available. What do you think will be the eventual outcome of the victim of that sudden cardiac arrest?

Medical first responders are often the first to respond and render aid to an emergency medical assistance call. The idea, or concept of medical first responders, came about mostly because paramedic units or even basic ambulances are just too costly to put in enough places to help each and every citizen that has an accident or falls ill fast enough.

Medical First Responders can be, and about half of the time are, volunteers. What type of MFR you will encounter, or which one will come to your aid, usually depends on whether you find yourself in an urban area or rural area. In less densely populated areas, you can expect that the local volunteer fire department or the county road patrol will have the responsibility to be the designated MFR's. In the urban or inner city areas, it is most of the time, the local police or full-time professional fire departments who act in this role.

Whoever they are, and whatever organization they may be attached to, they are an indispensable part of our success in saving lives and reducing mortality and morbidity. The vast majority of MFR's are there to help in any way that they can. They do everything from cardiopulmonary resuscitation (CPR), being stretcher-bearers, or running for needed equipment. In fact, they are usually tripping over each other to be of some help. They like being "involved" and are almost always willing to do anything to help, no matter how trivial it may seem to the casual bystander.

The professional MFR's are members of full-time fire or police departments that have received training in emergency first-aid, CPR, and in the use of an automatic, external defibrillator (AED). However, those who are members of full-time professional fire departments are at times a little different than those who come from volunteer departments. The difference is experience and repetition.

The full time men and women usually have more opportunities to put their skills to use. The number of times the full time MFR's have to practice their skills in "real life" situations, the more proficient and comfortable they become. That's not to say they don't get a little flustered and anxious at times. They do. For instance, many MFR's think that all chest pain must be heart related.

During one call, a cop got a little excited when he thought that we weren't in a big enough rush for this 30-year-old female with "chest pain". He was just sure her chest pain meant that she was having a major heart attack. There she was, on the couch, thrashing about and rolling around like she's on fire or some such thing. The cop had her lying down, with her feet in the air. The problem is, when people are suffering real cardiac pain or are in cardiac distress of any kind, there is almost always a respiratory component.

Breathing adequately becomes a concern with respiratory rate, tidal volume, and gas exchange. Lying flat on your back with your feet in the air inhibits each of those three mechanisms. Consequently, it's the exact opposite of what is needed when you think that someone is having a cardiac event.

We found out later that the woman was just upset over some personal issue she was having with her boyfriend and now all hell was breaking loose. It was more drama than a medical issue. When I first arrived and ruled out the possibility of a heart related problem, I thought that she might be experiencing an anxiety attack. Those are real events that shouldn't be minimized in their ability to disable someone during the brief time of their psychological crisis. But it wasn't even that.

Don't misunderstand; I don't blame the police officers for not knowing the difference. They're not supposed to differentiate between what is real and what is (in this case) a drama queen. He felt more relaxed when we informed him that the lady he thought was possibly having a heart attack, in fact wasn't having any such thing. The way she was rolling around, screaming, yelling, not answering questions, and in general just acting like a fool, he probably thought she would die before more help could arrive. I guess if I were in his situation I would be a little testy myself.

When it comes to volunteers one thing is certain, more often than not, they are a very passionate group of people that have their hearts in the right place. Over the years, I've grown to deeply appreciate the wide and vast majority of those that are MFR's. At the scenes of serious illnesses or accidents, there is always the need for more help. It seems that there are never enough hands to do everything that needs to be done. Sometimes you may need a firefighter to assist you in extricating somebody from a car that is wrapped around a tree, or help you carry a person down three flights of stairs. At another time, that same firefighter can be useful in just holding an IV bag.

On the other end of the spectrum, there are those who never quite seem to "get it." Too many times they offer unsolicited comments about what they "think" may be the proper or more appropriate course of treatment. For this reason, it's apparent to the professional EMS provider, that the MFR with this kind of mind set doesn't fit in. They appear clumsy, aloof, and are more times than not, in the way and counter-productive. At this end of the scale, they are more concerned with how many patches they have on their shirts, the crease in their pants, or how cool they look with a stethoscope hanging around their neck. And by all means let us not forget how important it is to know how big and bright the light bar is on their vehicle.

One example was this young man that wanted to be an MFR in the worst way. The problem was he just wasn't very good at understanding medical concepts and emergency first-aid reasoning; not to mention, this kind of work isn't for just anybody. Undeterred, he kept on trying and unfortunately failing. The instructor finally decided that she'd had enough. After one class session she informed the individual that because he wasn't meeting the minimum standards, he was being released as a member of the instructional program. He vehemently argued her decision.

She responded, "Listen to me. You are only getting two out of every three answers to the questions I pose to you correct. So let me ask you this, if you only do things correctly on the scene of an emergency at a rate of two out of every three times, could you live with that?"

Without missing a beat, he says, "I don't have a problem with that!"

Luckily for everyone concerned (or those that may become concerned), the instructor said, "Well, I have a big problem with it and you're gone!"

Fortunately, those types of guys are few and far between. However, sometimes when the planets are properly aligned and the moon is almost full, those types of individuals do get into whatever organization that acts as first responders for medical emergencies. Eventually they will make a decision or initiate some kind of care that will leave you scratching your head in bewilderment.

I was once dispatched to a car versus train accident. Understandably, this kind of call gets everybody's juices flowing. Let's face it; the chances of there being death and destruction, not to mention incredible injuries, are really high. My partner and I were about twelve miles away when we received the call. When we arrived, the police and fire department personnel were already on the scene.

I immediately asked the officer, "How many people are in the car?" Although our dispatcher would obtain that type of information, I always ask because the information may change and we may need another ambulance to assist.

"There is one man down," the officer replied. I never asked about the train crew. I figured that if a freight train hits a car, and unless the collision is seen by the train crew, they may not know how many people were in jeopardy.

The car was mangled to the point of almost being unrecognizable. I then asked the same officer, "Is the person dead? Where is he?" He pointed behind one of the three fire trucks on the scene. We drove the ambulance right up to where the victim was laying and saw several people standing in a circle. As I got out of the ambulance, I could see that somebody was doing chest compressions. I was immediately aghast with disbelief!

Two or three guys from the all-volunteer fire department were taking turns doing CPR on a middle-aged man who was just about cut in half. He was ripped open across his entire abdomen, right below his rib cage. Most of his abdominal organs were smashed and leaking out of both sides of his torso. On top of that, blood was squirting out of the victim's mouth and nose during each chest compression. Without a doubt, he was incredibly dead.

"What in the hell are you doing, and why are you assaulting that corpse?" I yelled.

Again, without missing a beat the one doing the compressions retorts, "We're doing CPR! What does it look like?"

In a highly critical tone I said to him, "It appears to me that you all made a poor decision!"

As providence would have it, a medical doctor that I knew fairly well, just happened to be driving by. He saw all of the commotion and stopped to see if he could be of some assistance. He was of great assistance, but not for the reasons he thought he would be. I stood at the back of the ambulance with the back doors open, pissed off, and getting ready to pull out the cot to transport the victim to the hospital.

The doctor tapped me lightly on the shoulder and said, "Need any help, fella?"

I said, "Oh Doc, am I ever glad to see you here. Hey, I need your help in calling this one. Some putz started CPR on a profoundly dead guy!"

The doctor asked me to show him. As he made it through the crowd of onlookers he grimaced. He just turned to me and softly said, "You can call this one, Jim."

I thanked him and told him that if my partner and I would have been here first, we were certain that we would not have started any kind of life-saving measures. He shook his head in agreement, walked back to his car, and drove away. There was not a single complaint from any of the volunteer MFR's. I'm sure after they got into this one particular event, and as they were doing CPR, they probably came to the inevitable realization of their folly. It is just a small example of not thinking before acting.

But because train versus car accidents are luckily very rare events, it is easy to understand how volunteers in particular will get a little overwhelmed in their thought processes. It's mostly because you know on the way to the call, that it is in all likelihood going to be a hell of a mess and there will be people critically hurt and most likely, dead.

***

Another time that sound reasoning seemed to be left at the station, was when the emergency call came of a house fire. We go to watch over the firefighters and to lend medical treatment if necessary. When we arrived, the house was fully engulfed; fire was coming out of nearly every window.

As I was just standing beside one of the fire trucks watching the dozen or so men battle the blaze, there was some talk of perhaps someone being in the house. At the moment, it was really nothing more than a rumor started by a couple of the neighbors who didn't know the whereabouts of the occupant of the house.

One of the firefighters started stomping around, then got mad about one thing or another before he decided he must mount a rescue effort. When I saw just how intent he was, I thought, *Oh man, you've got to be kidding me!*

So I approached the firefighter and grabbed the guy by the sleeve of his coat and said, "Hey man, I don't mean to tell you what to do or anything like that, but what are you thinking? You can't get within a hundred feet of that blazing inferno without wearing fire equipment, and it's been a blaze like this for at least the last twenty minutes that I've been here. I assure you if there was anybody in that house, they're well beyond your help now. Do me a favor and don't kill yourself."

He looked at me in anger but didn't say a word. He just jerked his sleeve out of my hand and continued to stomp around. Some of the other firefighters saw our brief encounter. They notified the fire chief who quickly put a stop to what would certainly be a very dangerous and really foolish endeavor. As it turned out, there wasn't anybody in the house. The homeowner was in fact out at a local bar at the time; she didn't even know that her house was on fire.

While some MFRs can be hasty, the vast majority that I routinely encounter are of immense help and assistance. Even an ordinary citizen can be invaluable and indispensable in a critical situation. More times than not, everyday people will extend themselves in remarkable ways when they see someone in distress and in need of the type of help that simply cannot wait.

Almost as serious as a car versus train accident, is a call that a plane has gone down. We got such a call. We received an emergency call that a plane had gone down along the St. Joseph River. The long winding river starts in northwest Indiana and twists its way through most of Berrien County in southwest Michigan before emptying into Lake Michigan. It is heavily covered in most places with trees along its winding path. Apparently a plane went down by the river but nobody could find it. The local police and fire departments were activated but didn't really know where to go.

As we headed to the general location, I had what turned out to be a relatively good idea. My dad is a pilot and owns a small plane called a Piper Cub. Those planes were built and used during World War II for reconnaissance purposes. I called him and told him that a small plane went down in the Eau Claire area and the emergency services couldn't find it. We didn't know how many people were on board or anything in particular.

I said, "Can you get in the air and find it? We don't really know where to look."

Dad had been a firefighter and captain of the all-volunteer Bridgman City Fire Department for a number of years. Although he had retired from the fire department he always extended himself to help. "I'll be right there. Just watch for my signal!" he hung up the phone before I could ask what the signal would be.

I called back right away, but my mother said he ran like hell out of the house, grabbed my brother John (who is also a pilot), and they both ran into the airplane hanger that was in the back yard. Within four to five minutes, I saw Dad's plane fly right by us. I was really proud to see him coming to the aid of a fellow pilot. Most of the private aviators know each other and are friends, so he already had a vested interest in assisting EMS and the local fire department in their rescue efforts.

Once our ambulance arrived at the staging point designated for this rescue, I jumped out of the ambulance and told personnel from the sheriff's department, local police, and fire departments that the plane in the air was my dad's. I told them that I had taken it upon myself to call them into action to be of assistance, and that they would find the downed plane for us. About a minute or so later, Dad pointed the right wing sharply toward the ground and started a tight circling pattern.

When I saw that I yelled, "That's it! That's where the plane is! He found it! He found it!"

My partner Ed Witucki and I quickly jumped back into our

ambulance and drove it across a big cornfield, taking down at least two rows of corn at a time. We couldn't see anything other than corn stalks flying all around us. I remember thinking that we must look like the fastest combine in the world, going through this cornfield at probably forty miles per hour. There were corn stalks stuck in our front bumper, side view mirrors, and even our light bar.

Sure enough, Dad led us right to the downed plane. As soon as we arrived on scene, they flew off and went back home. The other emergency units followed us and we came to the assistance of one man in the plane. As we scrambled up onto the wing in an attempt to get the door of the low winged airplane open, Ed noticed that several treetops were sheared off. He was right. The cockpit took a beating.

After we got the door open, we found a man that appeared to be in his mid-fifties unconscious, but still alive; however, he had sustained some massive head injuries. His eyebrows were pushed back into his head by approximately two inches. With the assistance of the firefighters, Ed and I got the pilot extricated and whisked him off to the closest hospital three miles away. Unfortunately, the pilot passed away two hours later. Everyone had done their level best—including my dad and brother. It was just yet another example of people stepping up to the plate and coming to the aid of somebody in need.

In another incredible incident where volunteers working as medical first responders were truly heroic, was during a call to the local state park on Lake Michigan. All too frequently there are people there who don't have any respect for the many dangers that the Great Lakes can pose, and they succumb to the several drownings—or near drownings annually. On this particular day, our call was to rescue a 9-year-old boy from Ohio. He and his family were there for the weekend. The young man came up missing and was found about fifteen minutes later floating facedown in the lake.

When the volunteers from the Lake Township Fire Department arrived, the boy was in cardiac arrest. The firefighters and park rangers immediately started CPR, and when my partner and I arrived about eight minutes later nothing much had changed in the young man's condition. I quickly intubated the patient so we could better ventilate him. My partner hooked him up to our cardiac monitor and we defibrillated him two or three times before we got him converted into a sustained cardiac rhythm.

We established an IV and finally got him stabilized. All of this was done right on the beach sand, in front of the boy's parents and siblings. When I first announced to the other rescuers that we just got his pulse back, his father said, "Thank God," and he began to cry. The boy's mother was just in a state of shock. I think you could have thrown a bucket of ice water on her and she probably wouldn't have noticed at all. She was in such a mental shutdown that she actually looked catatonic. She was absolutely and completely unemotional.

As we were about ready to transport the boy to the hospital eighteen miles away, he started to take a few breaths on his own. That's always really good news. I told the boy's father that his son was starting to breathe a little bit, and although he was a long way from being out of the woods, that things were indeed looking up. As I was talking with his father, my partner continued to assist the boy in breathing by mechanical means. The firefighters and park rangers who started the rescue efforts in the first place, removed our patient from the beach, and loaded him into the back of the ambulance. As long as I shall ever live, I never will forget the look on the father's face, or forget what he said.

With all of the passion and humility any human can convey, he simply stated, "How can I thank you? I owe you my life."

I instantly felt a lump in my throat and I gently replied to him, "You don't owe me a thing. If you want to thank some very deserving people, thank those firemen and park rangers; they're the bunch that saved your son. Had it not been for them, your boy wouldn't be alive right now. The only thing I did was to continue what they had started. Without them, it would not have made any difference whether or not paramedics like me were here at all."

With tears streaming down his face, he just shook his head in acknowledgement and mustered up one more heart felt, "Thank you."

As I climbed into the back of the ambulance, I don't know whether or not he had a chance to say anything to the five or six volunteer firefighters and park rangers who were there as medical first responders. I thought at the time that the best thing for our patient was to have both my partner and me in the back of the ambulance with him. The reasoning was to more closely monitor him during our expeditious, twenty-five minute ride to the nearest emergency department. In twenty minutes, with a very critical patient, things can go from bad to worse, and back again with amazing speed. He needed to have two paramedics attending to him.

One of the firefighters volunteered to drive us to the hospital and we were off like a shot. During our rapid trip, the condition of our patient continued to improve as he opened and closed his eyes every so often, moved a little bit, and started to fight the endotracheal tube that we had inserted into his airway earlier. We arrived safely at the hospital without further incident and turned our patient over to the eagerly awaiting, and highly competent emergency room staff.

Days after the call, I saw some of the MFR's who came to the boy's rescue. They inquired about how he was doing and about his expected prognosis. I told them that he was awake and alert (still in the hospital) and things were really looking up. One of the guys said with really no excitement in his voice, "Hey, that's great."

The other guy picking up on the first guy's comment said, as he was sipping a cup of coffee, "Yeah, that's really good news."

And that was about all there was to their curiosity. No beating of their chests, no self-congratulations, no thinking they're bigger than life. Those types of volunteers and MFR's are the best. They see a need in their communities and take it upon themselves to fill it. They acquire the necessary training and continue to do what they have been taught—to give 110%. For the communities in which they serve, they are in fact absolutely indispensable. For me, they are truly heroic.

Chapter 4
THE WORST DAYS

The worst days in most any profession is where someone falls ill, is injured, or in the extreme, is killed. Those days are understandably catastrophic for all involved. In the profession of emergency medical services, coming to the aide and rescue of people that are either gravely ill or critically injured, are our best days. Because of that, EMS is unlike any other profession.

Most, if not all EMS workers (whether professional or volunteer) thrive and excel on those calls that are the most critical and life threatening. For me, it has not been unusual to have just completed a twenty-four-hour shift that was augmented by two cardiac arrests (one of which being a sudden infant death syndrome (SIDS) tragedy), a high-speed vehicular accident where one person was killed—and the other two ended up in surgical suites fighting for their lives—and a child victim of a near drowning.

When my aforementioned shift comes to a welcome end, I scan my timecard through the time clock, and head for the back door where my car awaits me in the employee parking lot. At long last I have a solitary moment to reflect and to contemplate what happened on such a shift. I marvel and question, why people like me flourish and stand out in a world filled with people that suffer untimely sudden death, and experience tremendous pain and injury? My conclusion is always the same...I don't have a clue.

As I speed homeward, I continue to think about all that I have seen, all that I have done. I wonder about lives cut short and those that ended before they hardly started. Although I feel regret for those lost lives, I tend to have more sympathy for those who do live, but may never fully heal. The empathy I sense for the family and friends of those taken too early is staggering. For me, the thought of a terrible and life-altering injury to one of my children or burying one of my children for whatever reason, is worse than any other possibility.

I think of that log sheet that gives a record of all of those patients and their families whose lives have been changed, possibly forever.

It bears witness to the pain and suffering of the victims and their families that, in the blink of an eye, became my patients. On my log sheet I see the events of the day that tell of the human carnage of really bad days for a few people. They went about their day thinking the sun would rise and set for them just as it always had. Little did they know, when they got out of bed that day, it would be their last. For decades I have observed the effects of sudden and unexpected death on families, and without exception, it is stunning and horrendous.

Most people may come to the logical conclusion that for the men and women of EMS, that these are the worst days. I'm here to tell you, that's not true. For EMS workers universally, those are the best days. We look back on days like this with a tremendous amount of satisfaction. We look to be at our best in coming to the assistance for those few people who are suffering their worst. Because of that pain and anguish we know that we truly made a difference between life and death for people in need of our care. We know that we reduced the suffering and personal sorrow for countless family members, friends, and colleagues of those who were victims, or were struck by a very real and personal tragedy.

Unfortunately, we also know of the frailty of the human condition, and that although we go out of our way to not get involved on any emotional level, we too succumb on that very rare occasion to the one call that tests your courage, professionalism, and humanity. We all know that each of us today will die in any number of tomorrows, and that we may die in any number of ways. As human beings, we don't care to think of our mortality or how we will spend our last day on the planet. It's clearly a thought and subject that is unsettling and disturbing.

The very nature of EMS means that I will face and be a part of someone's last day. I will face and be a part of the emotional trauma that elicits profound sadness, shock, confusion, and outright disbelief. It is inherent in the medical business at large that there is a built-in emotional defense mechanism that protects the men and women who are treating those that are either sick or injured from attaching themselves to their patients.

It is a defense mechanism that allows people like me to go to

work each and every day and do it for years without suffering—
too severely—the effects of a psychological trauma. I believe it is
God's way of helping those of us in EMS to be able to face the life-
altering illnesses of our patients, the senseless acts of violence,
and the inequality and sometimes the ruthlessness of humanity on
a daily basis.

For me, trouble arises when my defense mechanism fails for
whatever reason. There is no warning of it. There is no defense for
it. Even though I consider myself an emotional rock, there have
been those extremely rare occasions when I have found myself
being just as human as the next guy. It may be from a set of circumstances in the patient I see, which too closely reminds me of
someone in my family or a close friend with the same set of circumstances. It may be the patients themselves who trouble me.

For me, it is usually a very sick or badly injured child that
resembles in appearance or mannerism one of my three children.
Sometimes the only thing it may take is a touch, a glance, or a few
poignant words that cause my defenses to come tumbling down.
Fortunately, the vast majority of the time it's not an issue. However,
every so often, one ambulance call in several thousand will bother
me anywhere from a couple of weeks to several months.

One call has haunted me for years. Even though that "one"
call happened more than a dozen years ago, a healthcare worker
recently told me that because of that call, in her opinion, I suffered
from post traumatic stress disorder (PTSD). Usually (and outside of
this writing) I have attempted to tuck that incident away in a deep,
dark place in the back of my mind where only my life's demons
live. I continue to hope that in enough time it will fade or simply rot
away.

On my way to work (and for no particular reason) that one
ambulance call popped into my consciousness. In no time I find
myself praying that nothing I see today will remind me of that
once-in-a-career call that still grips me with fear, dread, loathing,
and lingering regret. The vast majority of the time the prayer is
granted. On rare occasion the answer is, "Sorry, you're the only
one available." Those are the times when I feel the most alone
and vulnerable. That's when I sense the weight of the world sitting

on my shoulders and when indecisiveness is tugging at my sleeve.

The following are a few short stories that are true events that caused me to pose a question to myself, "Can I go back to work tomorrow?"

***

I had only been working as a basic EMT for maybe a year in the summer of 1978 when we received an ambulance call along with the local police and fire departments. We were called to respond to a railroad crossing at the very northern edge of the township. A call had been received from somebody who reported that a freight train had just struck a car.

As you can imagine, a train versus car accident gets everybody's blood pumping. As for me, when I heard the dispatch for this potentially horrific accident, I felt a very tense and nervous excitement. As I ran out of my parent's house, jumped into my car, and sped my way to the ambulance station, I could feel my heart beating through my chest. I knew that as a basic EMT I would have more emergency medical training than anyone responding to this incident. I would be expected to lead the rescue or the recovery efforts. Knowing that, and understanding that my level of experience was still very limited, got my juices running.

Everybody dispatched knew that such a call for help meant the injuries were going to be really bad. And, they knew that death was more than just a possibility, it was a distinct probability. When I arrived, I saw that a heavily-loaded freight train had indeed collided with what I found out later was a brand new out of the showroom, Ford LTD.

As I got to the car, I heard the cries of what sounded like a woman. The car was upside down and lying in tall weeds. All of the windows had been shattered or blown out, and the car itself was just a mangled, almost unrecognizable wreck. Under it all was a woman lying flat on her back, fully conscious and aware of what had just occurred. Since I could only see just the one woman and nobody else, I immediately asked four or five of the volunteer firemen to check the perimeter of the car path in case others may have been in the car with her, and had been ejected along the way. She was alone.

Since rolling the car off of her could cause her more injuries or exacerbate the injuries she had already sustained, I decided that since there was also a tow truck on scene we would lift the car straight up and off of her. While the firemen were working at getting the tow truck driver close to the car, I was crawling under the car, introducing myself, and assuring her we would get her to the hospital as soon as possible. Two other firemen also were digging their way toward her to help assess her injuries.

What I found was shocking. Although she was lying flat on her back partially covered in dirt and broken glass, her hips were turned at a ninety-degree angle to her back. Her legs were turned yet another ninety degrees from her hips. Her particular injuries from her pelvis on down instantly reminded me of one of those cheap little dolls kids can turn so its legs are facing backwards.

Both of her legs and thighs had trauma-induced gross deformities with each angulated, and bent in several places that indicated many obvious fractures between her hips and her feet. She had a fractured pelvis, forearm, clavicle, and we later learned all of her ribs on her left side were fractured. When we were able to lift the car and slide a backboard under her, we needed to get her into the correct anatomical position. That meant that we needed to straighten her hips and legs.

As we were turning her onto the backboard, I can still vividly remember feeling the grating of her broken pelvis and each of the three leg bones grinding together. Throughout this ordeal, she was fully alert and aware of her surroundings and what had happened to her. Her pain although considerable, wasn't as bad as I thought it might be or should have been. I took this as an unmistakable sign of the early stages of shock. Although all of the rescuers were putting forth their best efforts, it still took us better than ten minutes to get her out from under her wrecked car.

Once we got her on the backboard, she told me she was getting dizzy. As I looked closely at her, I could see that she looked pale. I didn't know whether she was pale when I got to her side because the car that was lying on top of her was also shading just enough light to prevent us from seeing her skin clearly. Even though I was just an EMT with very limited field experience, I could see that her condition was rapidly deteriorating.

I spoke with her to keep her calm. "I'm going to put this oxygen mask on you and give you a lot of oxygen. I don't want you to fight it. It's what you need most right know."

Just as I was about to cover her mouth and nose with a non-rebreathing oxygen mask designed to deliver up to 100% oxygen, she looked at me with her eyes big, wide, and blazing with intensity. With a stern jaw, pursed lips, and panic in her voice she cried out, "I don't want to die! Jim, don't let me die! Don't let me die Jim!"

I remember telling my dad (who was one of the many firemen at the scene) that the way she looked at me and grabbed at me with her uninjured arm, she was literally scared to death. Somehow, I think she knew that she was hurt and broken to the point that she would most likely die. Over the years it's been my experience that people that truly believe they are going to die, almost always do.

During our rapid transport to the hospital, I splinted her legs as best as I could, mostly for her comfort. Other than giving her oxygen and having her back boarded and collared, splinting her legs was about all we could do other than to get her to the hospital as quickly as possible. At that time, there were no paramedics and therefore no pre-hospital advanced life support. We didn't even have medical anti-shock trousers (MAST) pants.

As she pleaded for her life, I remember her panicked cries raising my anxiety as well as the hair on the back of my neck, and her searing eyes just pierced my soul. In the nearly thirty years since that call, I've never seen anybody with eyes filled with so much terror. My father called me the next day and told me that she died of myocardial contusions. It was the first person I had treated as a patient that died from injuries sustained in a car accident. I felt strangely empty and I had a sense of loss that was unsettling.

Arriving at work the next day, I remember getting out of my car, putting my station key into the door lock, opening the door, entering the station, and the door slamming shut behind me. As the noise of that heavy steel door slamming echoed throughout the firehouse, I suddenly felt very small and mortal. Of course, we all know that our time on this earth is limited, but when you're 20 years old and healthy, who thinks about death? It was the first time in my life that the frailty and the uncertainness of tomorrow came to light.

Three days later, while at home mowing the front yard, somebody pulled into our driveway, walked up to the house, and knocked on our front door. After making a few laps around the yard with the mower, I happened to look up and I saw Dad and this other man standing on the driveway waiting for me to come around again with the mower. I shut the mower off, and before I said a word he immediately took a few steps into the yard, extended his hand to me, and said it was his wife who had been in the car accident. I was stunned.

At first, I thought that he might have had a complaint about something, or at least a concern about the way we handled the care of his wife. Instead, he couldn't thank me or the rescuers enough. As he started to talk, his voice was already cracking. After thanking me he was crying so hard I could barely understand him. He just told me how much he loved his wife, how she loved life, and how much he already missed her.

By the time he was finished, I felt so bad for him and his heartfelt loss that I nearly had tears running down my face as well. Up to this day, I have never seen a man bare his soul to me in such a way. He told me how much he would miss his wife's touch, her smile, and her kiss. To listen to him talk through his tears of love and now his love lost, was for me a truly remarkable and moving experience.

As I reflect on that particular call, I really marvel and am astounded at how that one call changed my life and how I think about life itself. Perhaps being nothing more than mortal, we're not supposed to understand why things happen as they do. Perhaps we just don't have the wisdom to understand the deeper meaning to life.

***

Shortly after I left Lake Township and started my current employment with Medic 1 Ambulance, it was yet to be another month before we would actually start applying what we had learned the year before. I punched the time clock for the first time at Medic 1, August 1, 1979. I finished my formal training and was licensed as a paramedic in the State of Michigan in November of 1978. It wasn't until a month after I started at Medic, that we would run our first ever pre-hospital, advanced life support call.

All of the paramedics who started the advanced life support program, me included, were only in our early twenties. Our classroom training had been successfully completed, and I guess the powers that be just thought that we would be starting up the paramedic ambulance shortly after we completed our training. To make matters worse, because of insurance issues and medical liability, we couldn't work in the emergency department anymore because we were no longer students. That meant that if we were lucky we were only going to be a little rusty in all of our skill levels! We had no mentors, and no one to take us under their wing and show us the way.

There were plenty of growing pains. In retrospect, who in their right mind would think that any of this was going to go smoothly, let alone error free? Looking back on that early time, it was plain to see that it was tailor made for mistakes and missteps. When I look back on it and think about what could have gone wrong, it's a wonder that we ever got the paramedic program off the ground at all.

One day after working twenty hours into our twenty-four-hour shift, my partner Dave Hawkins and I responded to assist one of our basic ambulance crews. It was 4 a.m., and they were on the scene of an elderly gentleman who was complaining of crushing chest pain and severe shortness of breath. When we arrived, the basic crew already had the patient on oxygen, had recorded all of his vital signs, obtained a medical history, and had his medicines ready for me to look at.

Dave quickly attached the cardiac monitor leads to the patient while I looked at his arms to start an IV. Did I mention that because there was no electricity in the house all of this was being done by the light of a laryngoscope blade? After finding a vein adequate for cannulation, I established the IV and then turned my full attention to the cardiac monitor to see what type of rhythm his heart was exhibiting. I quickly noticed that he was having several premature ventricular contractions (PVCs), which are dangerous. If they occur at a rate of twelve or more per minute, and if they originate from more than one spot in the ventricles, they may cause the heart to go into fibrillation.

As I zeroed in on the PVCs, I was consumed with the singular thought of suppressing that very dangerous dysrhythmia. What I didn't look hard enough for (and consequently didn't interpret correctly) was the underlying rhythm of his heart. Human hearts beat in what we call a normal sinus rhythm. It's the rhythm that is seen on the cardiac monitor and considered to be the way the heart is supposed to be sending the electrical impulses down through the heart.

His underlying rhythm was atrial fibrillation, which means that the top part of his heart was beating erratically or just plain quivering. And, the bottom part was beating normally, but usually irregularly. By itself, that type of heart rhythm is in the short term benign and is not considered dangerous. But if you add an irritable ventricle that is causing the heart to start a heartbeat from the bottom part of the heart or ventricle, and if there is more than one every five seconds, it's a problem. If those PVCs are coming from more than one spot in the ventricles, it's a big problem.

At that time the drug that we used most of the time to stop—or at the least curtail PVCs— was called Lidocaine. This anesthetic was used to anesthetize the heart muscle in order to take the irritability out of the muscle, to allow the heart to beat normally. It's a cousin to the drug Novocain, which is given by dentists to numb the mouth and gums.

As with any drug, there are times and circumstances when the medication I want to give to solve a problem may make matters worse, and therefore contraindicated. Lidocaine is not contraindicated in atrial fibrillation as long as my patient's heart is beating faster than sixty beats per minutes, as his was. About ten seconds after administering the drug, he looked at me without uttering a sound. He gave me this quizzical look, started to lose consciousness, and then started to have a seizure.

The rest of the guys held him down as I immediately looked at the EKG monitor. He was now in Ventricular Tachycardia (V-tach), a heart rhythm that happens when the ventricles of the heart start beating wildly. A heart rate of 220 beats per minute or higher is not unusual. The problem is that when the ventricles beat that fast, they don't have the time to fill with blood before the next heart beat. That causes a precipitous drop in blood pressure, which in turn causes very little blood to be circulated around to the vital organs.

The lack of adequate blood perfusion can cause amongst other things, death. The rhythm is considered not only highly dangerous, but also lethal. I instantly had two thoughts. First, "How can this be? This drug that I just injected into this man is supposed to prevent or suppress this type of rhythm!" Secondly, "Holy cow, did I just cause this?" I reached for the man's neck to check his pulse and found out quickly that although the man had a heart rhythm on the monitor, he had no discernable pulse, and therefore was in the process of dying. That's when the panic started.

The four of us were working a cardiac arrest instead of just some poor guy with chest pain and a little shortness of breath. Although I knew what to do and how to do it, I remember being in a daze and struggling just to keep focused on the task at hand. I gave him all of the necessary drugs, in the correct order, in the correct dosage, at the correct time, but no matter what I or my partner and the two guys from the other crew did, things just deteriorated to the point that his heart had completely stopped.

I intubated him, and we gave him more drugs, vigorous CPR and in the end, it just didn't matter. My patient died right then and there. We rushed him to the hospital and as I'm ventilating him and Dave is doing chest compressions, I was really bewildered and just emotionally crushed. Then Hawkins flippantly says to me, "Goddamn Stine, I don't think we ever killed one off until now!"

I could have smacked him right in the teeth for that comment. I probably would have if I didn't think that he just might be right.

After we arrived at the hospital with our patient, the emergency room staff did all they could to revive our patient, but he was gone. Dr. Small came up to me after he pronounced the patient dead and could plainly see that I was really upset.

"Jim, these are sometimes the unintended consequences of what we do," he said in an attempt to console me. What he said may have been true, but I will never forget the look on that man's face when he just faded from life.

***

I have to tell you that there was a time that treating badly injured or critical kids didn't bother me much—or at the least not more than any other call might have. That has since changed. I'm not sure when it changed, but it was probably when my first son was born. From the very moment I saw him in the delivery room, I was instantly and passionately in love with him. He was everything that I ever wanted. He was a big boy, weighing almost nine pounds, had big blue eyes, and blonde hair. He was absolutely perfect.

Today, my wife and I now have three grown children and three little grandsons. I earnestly hope and pray that I never have to bury any of them. The emptiness and hurt of such a loss is something that I hope to never experience. Kids do get hurt and they do fall ill. As a result, I treat them with many of the same techniques, as well as the same medicines and fluids, with which I treat adults.

When discussing the differences in circumstances of injuries and illnesses to adults and children, there are two rules that almost always apply. There are exceptions to these rules, but the difference is nearly always this: First, one way or another, adults almost always get what they deserve. Secondly, kids almost always are the innocent victims of an adult's poor decision.

What I mean is, adults choose to abuse alcohol and involve themselves in illicit drug use. Adults decides to drink and drive, or to drive recklessly and injure or kill themselves and others. Adults put themselves into dangerous situations with self-imposed inclusion of gang life, crime, and gun violence.

Kids who are in gangs, involved with crime and that lifestyle, are themselves victims of a parent's or an adult's neglect, indifference, and the lack of a quality family structure. So I have a real soft spot for kids of every race, creed and walk of life. It injures me to my soul to see kids banged up in car wrecks because they are not restrained properly with seat belts or car seats. It infuriates me to near insanity to see kids who are ill because of neglect or have sustained great emotional, mental or physical abuse.

Over the past thirty-five years in EMS, I have experienced some of the worst decisions adults made that led to a child being victimized by their folly.

***

My partner and I got dispatched to back up another ambulance on a car accident that had several victims. Some elderly gentleman (that probably had no business being behind the wheel of an automobile in the first place) came off of the local interstate highway and ran his pickup truck through the stop sign at the end of the exit ramp. He slammed his truck into the side of a car loaded with three small children, which careened into another car injuring two more people. Of course the 82-year old driver of the pickup had just a few minor cuts and bruises.

When I arrived, I immediately asked the first paramedic—who was still trying to sort things out—if he knew who was the most seriously injured? He told me that most everybody was okay, except for a 6-year-old boy who was apparently unconscious. I quickly ran to where he was being attended to by the first paramedic's partner.

This particular paramedic wasn't then very competent at all. He was kind of indecisive on how and what he wanted to do for his patient. About the only thing he had done in the three to four minutes before we arrived (and was still doing) was just assessing him. In that type of accident, that should take no more than twenty seconds. Does he have a pulse? Is he breathing? What is his level of consciousness? Are there any obvious injuries? That's it. That's all that is required initially.

So, I pulled rank and told him in a most stern tenor, to get his ass out of the way and get me a backboard, cervical collar, and to help my partner retrieve our ambulance cot. My partner and I quickly extricated the limp and unconscious little boy who was bleeding from his nose and one of his ears due to the impact of the pickup truck. Since all of the doors were jammed, we quickly slid the backboard through one of the broken windows, fitted him with a small cervical collar, and slid him onto the backboard. With great haste, we placed the backboard with our patient on it onto the cot and ran with it to our ambulance.

I remember looking down at this little boy and being incensed that he had not been in any car seat, or at the least a seat belt. As I looked down at him, he was exhibiting a decerebrate posture, which is exhibited by the victim of an acute traumatic brain injury. These victims' arms twist so the palms of the hands and the bottom of their feet are facing lateral. At that instant, I knew that his chances for a good outcome from his injuries were nil. Once inside the ambulance I remember tears running off the end of my nose, and yelling and screaming at the walls about why in the hell people can't put their kids in car seats or at the least seat belts.

Usually by this time I will have finished up with a more comprehensive assessment and treatment while my partner assisted the other crew or crews with their patients. This time, I told him that there would be no time to help anyone else; we needed to be at the hospital just as soon as humanly possible. Treating the patient, and a secondary assessment, would have to be done as we sped our way to the nearest medical facility.

I distinctly remember working feverishly on this little boy. My hands were just a blur with the speed of placing monitor leads on his chest, securing his airway through intubation, giving oxygen, starting an IV, and continuous assessment. All the while, I know that this little boy, through no fault of his own, was most likely fatally injured. Sadly, he did pass away the next day from skull and massive brain injuries.

***

One of the most profoundly sad, and at the same time one of

the angriest moments of my professional life, was one of the many cases of child abuse that I have witnessed first hand. This particular ambulance response was for a small girl that the caller reported wasn't breathing. At the time of this particular call I was working with my good friend and partner, Dave Nelson.

Dave is a big husky kind of guy that always likes to have a good time and always tries to find humor in just about everything he's involved in. He's also the kind of guy you want to see backing you up on an ambulance call when the proverbial excrement hits the fan. Unfortunately, Dave had to retire due to a medical disability a few years ago. Like many others, Dave was a very fine paramedic who knew what was important in EMS and what wasn't.

When the two of us received the call for the little girl not breathing, we were both asleep at our central station. As fast as we could, we scrambled out of the bunkroom, jumped into the ambulance, and blazed out of the station. We drove like hell and got to the scene of the emergency just as quickly as we could. When we first arrived, I grabbed our airway box and Dave grabbed our Life-Pak cardiac monitor. We both were "gloving-up" as we ran through the front door of the house. Three Benton Township police officers and a detective who were interviewing who turned out to be this little girl's grandfather.

We were immediately directed upstairs to the patient and bolted up the many steps where another officer was standing over the 6 year old who was laying on a throw rug next to her grandparent's bed. We didn't need much more than the light of the dimly lit bedroom to tell us that this little girl had been dead for at least an hour—and perhaps as long as three hours.

Because of the low lighting, it was impossible to see what had actually happened to her. The only thing we knew for sure was that because she was very cold to the touch, pulseless, and her eyes were fixed, dilated and glazed over, she was in fact, dead. Neither of us knew whether she had a medical condition that led to her death, or if she had somehow died of a choking accident, fall, or head injury. Kids do get into things that can often end in all kinds of trouble when they are not being properly monitored.

We went back downstairs to find out from the grandfather just what happened. As the police officers questioned him, he made mention that he disciplined her for something. His exact words were, "I want to be straight with you guys. I whooped her good!" We later found out that the mind-boggling reason for what turned out to be her last beating, was that she put her cartoon character slippers on the wrong feet.

Dave and I assumed an ambulance hadn't been called sooner because her grandfather may not have noticed that she had stopped breathing. After what turned out to be her last beating, she simply laid down next to her abuser's bed and quietly died from her injuries.

I couldn't imagine what might have gone through her little mind as she just breathed her last breath. When I attempt to put myself in those kinds of circumstances and try to imagine what it must have been like for her, I find it all but impossible. Not many of us can really and truly imagine and interpret what it must be like to get beaten and beaten until you simply…die.

It was fortunate for Dave and me (and certainly for the grandpa) that we didn't know two of the four officers present very well. I would be less than honest if I didn't say that Dave and I hadn't entertained thoughts of just kicking the hell out of this guy and then have him taken to jail. After the police had finished taking their pictures, and concluded their investigation, Dave and I got the okay from the county coroner to go ahead and move her body to the local hospital morgue.

The Benton Township chief of police at the time was a really good guy by the name of James Coburn. Chief Coburn met Dave and me, along with the medical examiner, and the detective at the little girl's house, at the morgue. In the morgue, there are bright fluorescent lights. Once we were able to get a really good look at her, I was shocked at what I saw.

The bright lights showed that this girl had dozens and dozens of scars. Through those bright lights a shadow was lifted that told the story of a girl whose life was almost entirely shrouded with one beating after another, after another. Some of her scars were deep, others superficial. She had scars that were new and others that were perhaps months or even years old.

But the thing that just about made me sick was this. When Dave and I first saw her (with a dimly lit incandescent light bulb) lying on that throw rug, we just thought that this little African-American girl had a very dark complexion. It wasn't until we saw her again in the morgue that what we thought was just the amount of melanin in her skin was in fact almost total body wide bruising.

Once we found parts of her that weren't beaten and heavily bruised, we were able to see that she actually wasn't all that dark. It was one of those times that your mind really doesn't believe what your eyes are telling it. At first I thought that she might have even had a skin condition that may have caused the discoloration. The medical examiner said that what we were witnessing, was in fact, massive, body-wide bruising.

My first words were, "That dirty bastard!"

Dave turned to Chief Coburn and said, "Jim, I want five minutes with that son-of-a bitch, right now!"

Of course that didn't happen. Dave and I were just as pissed off as we could possibly be and we were just blowing off some steam. I do ponder what may have happened at the scene of that most brutal of crimes if either Dave or I would had realized there instead of at the hospital, just how badly she was brutalized. I then think about our boss coming down to the county jail to bail us both out. I can assure you, neither the grandpa getting his ass kicked, nor the ass chewing from our boss, would have been pretty.

A few weeks later, I was called to testify for the prosecution for the murder of this poor little girl. I remember sitting on the witness chair testifying on what I saw, what I did, and most importantly what I heard. I told the prosecutor that I had heard the grandfather tell all of us that he "whooped her good."

"Mr. Stine, in your opinion, did he do that?"

While looking right at the jury, I said, "Yes sir. He certainly did."

At that moment about a third to half of the jury were squirming in their chairs. I was glad to see that. After all of the testimony, the grandfather was found guilty of second-degree murder and sentenced to a minimum of forty years in prison. Personally speaking, if I had been the presiding judge, I would have sentenced him to five minutes with Dave Nelson.

***

For me, the most awful and the most terrible call was the time that my partner and longtime friend Tim Zeneng, responded to a 9-1-1 call. This particular call was back in the mid 1980s, but is a call that will live with me in one degree or another, forever.

At the time of our dispatch, Tim and I were just sitting around watching TV at one of our outlying stations. The call came in as an assist to one of our nearby all-volunteer ambulance services for a child with a severe burn. When we received the address and started en route, we didn't know whether the burns were from heat from a house fire, a kitchen stove, or what. We didn't even know whether it was from a petroleum or chemical product, or even an electrical accident.

As we were speeding to the adjoining township, we received a call from one of the volunteer EMT's on scene that a young child and her uncle had been burned while raking leaves. The tone of his near-frantic voice told us that they were dealing with at least one critical patient, if not two very serious burns. It was obvious to the both of us that they needed advanced life support as soon as possible.

It took Tim and me only about six minutes to reach our desti-nation. Once we arrived, we were told that a 6-year-old girl was helping her uncle rake leaves when the gasoline he used to assist in the burning spilled on her; catching her clothing on fire. Appar-ently, she was kicking some smoldering leaves when her pant leg caught on fire.

According to her older brother, who happened to witness the entire event, the girl leaned over to pat the flames out with her gloved hands when the gas tainted gloves abruptly erupted in flames. From there, the flames rapidly spread to her light jacket and in just a few seconds her whole body was engulfed with flames. Her uncle stated that he was on the other side of the yard when he first heard his nephew yelling and his niece screaming for help. By the time he reached his niece and was able to extinguish the flames, he too was on fire.

The moment we arrived, there were policemen directing us where we were urgently needed. One of the volunteer EMT's came running around from behind his ambulance carrying the badly burned little girl in his arms. I was stunned when I saw just how extensive and massive the burns were on this little lady. Just looking at her for the first two or three seconds, I was in disbelief and aghast of what I was now witnessing. It was without out a doubt, the worst thermal burn I have seen in severity and scope with someone still alive.

In an instant, I had two thoughts. The first thought was that this little girl—through no fault of her own—was fatally burned and that there was going to be absolutely no way for her to survive this terrible accident. My second thought was that I wanted out of this. During these two instant thoughts, you just keep doing the best you can with the circumstances at hand.

So Tim and I quickly placed her on our cot inside the ambulance, and started to work. We instantly placed an oxygen mask over her little face and looked for a site where we might be able to start an IV. After looking for a minute or two, it was plain to see that since her burns were so extensive that IV cannulation at a peripheral level would be all but impossible.

Since we had just put her on oxygen, about the only thing we could do would be to maintain her airway, and rush her to the nearest hospital about twenty miles away. At that moment, Tim and I both felt pretty helpless. He did an outstanding job consoling the little girl and telling her that we were there to help her, and that she would be okay (knowing full well that his patient was doomed). Tim was always great with kids. It's a shame he never had any of his own. He would have made a great father.

Since there was not much that either of us would be able to do, I begged off the call and went to help the girl's uncle— a decision that I would regret for a long, long time. Tim told me he would be able to handle it and that I should attend to our other patient.

When I got out of our ambulance, the EMT's and other MFR's were just wheeling this guy on their cot up to their ambulance. I exited our ambulance with our drug box in hand ready to help the uncle. As I approached him, I noticed that although he had some severe second-degree burns and perhaps some third-degree burns, he would certainly recover from his injuries, unlike his niece.

As I was assessing his airway, giving him oxygen, and looking to start an IV, it was plain to see that he was clearly distraught. He kept inquiring of his niece's condition and what I thought about her chances of survival. I told him that his niece was critically burned (although I knew in my heart and mind that it would no doubt be fatal), and that he should pray for the best and prepare for the worst.

His treatment was relatively simple and straightforward. About the only thing to do for him was to figure the degree and percentage of surface area burned, start an IV for re-hydration, control his pain, and assess any pulmonary difficulties or changes in his breathing status. As I was started the saline IV and gave him oxygen, I had his niece on my mind. It bothered me that I pawned the little girl off on Tim; not because Tim would be inadequate on the little girl's treatment, far from it.

My mind told me at the time that there was very little that EMS could do in light of the magnitude and severity of the burns she sustained. My heart however, said I should have been at her side, not Tim. With the most critical of situations, I am always the paramedic that has had and welcomed the mantle of responsibility. I have always been the type of paramedic who takes and treats the most seriously injured patient.

Almost immediately I regretted that I didn't stay with that little girl. It should have been me that made absolutely sure that every little thing that could be done for her, was done. It should have been me that made sure that any and all measures to be taken to ensure her comfort would be taken. But I didn't.

I thought about myself first instead of my patient. I thought in an instant of the pain any dad (or uncle) would have knowing that he just burned his daughter to death in a terrible, but totally avoidable accident. I thought in an instant that it would be a pain that I couldn't tolerate at all. I thought in an instant that I wanted no part of it; even if it meant that someone else would be administering the care that I knew full well I should be giving.

For a long time after the incident, I felt like I let that little girl down by not being at her side. Although Tim would certainly do everything that I would do for her (and did), I still felt that I should have been there. At that moment in time I felt like a coward. After all, I did something that I hadn't done before, then, or for that matter since. I thought of myself before I thought of my patient.

Due to the nature of this horrific accident and the stresses it put on all of the medical first responders, firefighters and EMS personnel, the powers that be initiated a Critical Incident Stress Debriefing (CISD) a week after the call. It's the type of meeting that is open to anyone who had anything to do with a particular call that was particularly stressful or bothersome for whatever reason.

I have been on many, many calls in my more than thirty-five years in EMS that had warranted and received a CISD meeting. I never thought that a tough guy like me needed that sissy stuff. I thought that if you couldn't stand the pressure, you ought to get out of the EMS business. That call changed me forever in a number of ways.

Never again would I think that CISD would be for people that were a little too weak-kneed for EMS. Never again would I ever bail out of a call like I did with that little girl that day. She deserved better from me that day. She deserved the best I could possibly give and instead I gave her nothing. Instead I thought of myself and my articulated pain. Yes, she deserved better from me in her final hours on this planet, and I let her down.

During the CISD meeting there were about a dozen or more people there that had a hand in the call. My boss at the time, Bill Gebhard was there as well. I told everyone what I thought and finally what I did—or rather didn't do. I just sobbed. I just couldn't forgive myself for not being at her side during her trip to the hospital. To this day, that remains for me, the most excruciatingly horrendous call that I had ever experienced.

For a full eighteen months after that call, I went through a very personal hell each and every time I had to handle a critical pediatric patient. Each and every time I would just about come unhinged when I thought it might be up to me to actually have to really save a kid's life. Whether it was from a high velocity trauma, a near drowning, or a baby that had been victimized by SIDS, I went through my own emotional trauma every time I would respond to that type of call.

I remember very vividly, just trying in vain to sit still in the passenger's seat of the ambulance while the driver sped our way to any call that involved a youngster who was seriously ill or badly injured. I remember just squirming in my seat and saying to myself, *Oh God! Oh God! Please God, help me get through this.*

Of course in an instant, the all-too vivid memory of that little girl would be right there in front of me. Each time I would think about how I abandoned her, and the guilt of not staying with her, would just eat at me. Sometimes it took hours for me to shake that feeling. In my mind's ear, I could almost hear her say to me, "You let me down. You let me down." Like I said, it was at least eighteen months of sheer torture for me. Until this writing, I hadn't shared these thoughts with anybody.

I still think and wonder about that little gal. I think about how much her mother and father must still miss her. I think about how old she would be now if it weren't for that awful, awful accident. I think about all of the wonderful, and not so wonderful things that life would have had in store for her. At times I think maybe someday, in some way, I'll get the chance to tell her just how sorry I still am for failing her that fateful day.

Chapter 5
FAILURE: NOT AN OPTION

It's been my experience that the regular or standard EMS hourly shift is usually twelve or twenty-four hours long. During that time span there may be days that vary wildly as far as the severity of emergencies. We are dispatched and respond to everything from the, "Help me; I've fallen and I can't get up!" type of call, to the true traumatic or critical medical emergency call.

I've found (although this is far from scientific):

* 70% of the time, just about anybody with a standard First-Aid card can do what is needed for the patient at hand. That's about the number of "old fossil" basic life support transfers we do from nursing homes or adult foster care facilities, to any one of the local hospitals. It's usually because one of the local understaffed and overworked nursing homes is just now noticing that aunt Martha is now slobbering out of the left side of her mouth instead of her usual right side. And for whatever reason, today is the day we just have to find out why this is happening.

Unfortunately it also includes those taxi-cab calls that we are forced to respond to where the caller (usually a Medicaid recipient) "uses" EMS for simple transportation for such calls as minor scrapes and the ever present: "cough and cold that I've had for four days, and now at 3 a.m. it's somehow an emergency, and by God now I need an ambulance to drive my good-for-nothing sorry ass to the local hospital emergency room."

* 20% of the time, as the signs and symptoms of an injury or illness become more apparent, our emergency calls may require the level of someone trained in advanced first-aid or at the level of a basic EMT.

* 7% of the time will require the services of a highly-trained paramedic.

* 2% of the time will need that paramedic to not only have a high level of advanced life support training, years of experience and know-how, but will need that paramedic to be on top of their game at that particular moment.

* 1% of the time the patient (as well as the paramedic) will need

divine intervention (for those types of patients you wouldn't have bet a nickel on their survival, but they end up doing very well).

Some of the people who get into EMS do so by thinking they are there to save the planet and put funeral homes out of business. In no time at all, most of those same people come to the realization that reducing morbidity and not mortality, is what really occurs more than 95% of the time in those few patients who actually need pre-hospital advanced life support intervention. They also come to the understanding that death is going to find a way to eventually remove each of us from this world.

Consequently, I don't get too excited if I respond to a facility or a private residence where I find out that "Grandpa Jones," who is in his 92nd year, was found not breathing while lying in bed, where he had slowly been wasting away for the last several years. As Grandpa is busy breathing his last, the family is becoming excited and agitated over the situation.

But that's frequently the case where people are sometimes not prepared for the thought of life without 'ole Granddad. Sometimes it's because it's too uncomfortable to think about, or it's too much to deal with, or the thought of "we thought we had plenty of time to take care of that later." Occasionally people just don't realize how ill loved ones may be, or they are in denial about 'ole Granddad's health.

Finally, there are those few who are either in irrational denial or are just too dumb to understand, that in some cases, death can be expected at almost any time. No matter what the "or's" are, most people who call an ambulance for a loved one who is chronically ill, are not prepared for that particular death. That's not to say that I think people don't care whether their loved ones are living or have been slowly fading for many months or years. What I'm saying is that Grandpa's loved ones should care more about the last wishes and in the quality of life in Grandpa's fading years. To that end, a little more thought ought to be put forward as to the wishes and desires of all of those Grandpa's out there who are newly deceased or where death appears imminent.

Too many times we are called to help and to do "everything possible" to resuscitate old Uncle Hank. Too often those who are calling for EMS to help Uncle Hank are friends or relatives that have no idea of the general health and quality of life that may be an everyday struggle. They may know nothing of the specific malady that uncle Hank suffers from. As a result, they frequently react on emotion alone. All too often we respond to a call where end of life decisions have been made by the patient and still within the patient's immediate family there is crying, screaming, yelling, and gnashing of the teeth over whether we should be attempting to extend or prolong life. At this moment there is little thought of advanced directives that have been decided by either the patient, or the particular family member who is charged with legal power, to decide the medical matters which are pertinent to the care of Uncle Hank.

Because of this emotion-driven chaos, we as EMS providers may unwillingly force a gravely and terminally ill patient to die twice. Once, at the time of initial resuscitation, and the secondly when calmer heads and rational minds prevail to let nature take its course. At the moment of death, or where death appears inevitable, is certainly not the time where resuscitation efforts should be discussed with the immediate family, let alone be decided.

I don't get excited at all when I see the aforementioned Grandpa Jones or Uncle Hank lying on their deathbeds. I happen to think it's a blessing when Grandpa Jones or whoever can just fade away from life as we know it, surrounded by the love and affection of their family and friends. If they and their families are fortunate, there will be a lifetime of memories and stories for those who are left behind, and hopefully a legacy that can be cherished for generations.

What I as a professional paramedic get energized about and find as the ultimate life and death challenge, is the 12-year-old drowning victim, or the 22-year-old car accident victim, or the 32, 42, or 52-year-old heart attack victim. I get energized when the lives of many people will be altered and not for the better, if death or severe disability comes to the person I have been called to help. Those are the "or's" that get everybody in EMS animated, and they are the "or's" that bring out the best in the best paramedics.

Think about it, if the medical first responder and advanced life support crews are able to respond in a timely manner, and if they are able to do all of the skills that may be required, then the life that is saved may mean a life that is saved for many decades. That's why I don't get too wound-up with Grandpa Jones passing away in his 92nd year. And it's precisely why I do get intense if 12-year-old little Tommy is found floating face down in the family's swimming pool.

There have been countless times over the years when any one of my many partners and I have arrived at the scene of a life-threatening emergency, we have found that the family is in a full-tilt meltdown. Suddenly, something unexpected happens to someone in the nuclear family. Usually, it's Dad (or at least the father figure) that has suffered some sort of medical emergency. Many times over the years, I've entered a house where the dad had just collapsed or was so medically compromised that death could occur at any moment.

Sometimes a police or fire department medical first responder unit will be at the scene of the emergency a few minutes before we arrive. Shortly thereafter, we arrive with the ambulance with all of the advanced life support equipment on board to offer definitive care. Sometimes medical first responders aren't called or don't arrive in a timely manner, and we're the first ones to arrive. Whoever is first will almost invariably arrive to varying degrees of concern, chaos, and panic.

In the case where a dad has experienced a severe medical emergency, you will probably encounter the wife or mother of the family. She will be struggling, but doing her best to keep her emotions under control; often for the sake of her children who are screaming and crying. Depending on their ages, they may not know or understand why Dad's face is turning various shades of red, blue, or purple. Many times, the mom is straining to keep her composure to answer the necessary questions that EMS personnel have to ask. These questions may aid in her husband's treatment, and be critical to his very survival.

It is at this time where the mental and emotional strength of the EMS providers must come to the forefront. It is essential that we focus on the task at hand. It is also important to understand that while we have the immense responsibility of the critical care of the patient, we also have to get everybody around to work for, and with us.

Family members often feel helpless, so it's vital that to get them to do something. That may mean finding and retrieving medicines, moving furniture, clearing a walkway, or helping one of the medical first responders carry emergency medical equipment. Sometimes it means keeping another family member under control and out of everyone's way.

The following are a few true accounts of such emergencies where what we did as emergency care providers made all the difference. It was in those relatively rare times that failure to save a life, prevent, or help to minimize a severe disability, meant absolutely everything to someone. It's where failure was not an option.

***

One of the more remarkable, and certainly memorable calls that I was proud to have been a part of, was an early morning call that we had in a local village. Paramedic Ryan Cronk (one of my best friends) and I were both on duty. At approximately 6 a.m., we were awakened by our dispatcher and told that a 30-year-old man was having chest pain.

At first I was really irritated. Usually when someone calls because they or someone around them is having chest pain, the person assumes, and has been socially conditioned through the mass media, to think that it's heart related. It's safe to say that about 99% of the time when someone who is 30 years old, in generally good health, has no prior medical history of heart problems, but now has chest pain, it's a good bet it's because they were out partying the night before, and they have been vomiting most of the early morning hours away.

If they state that they have not imbibed in adult beverages, then there may be any number of other maladies. Chest muscle spasms, lung infection, cough, cold, pneumonia, or gastrointestinal distress may be a few of the more common and non-traumatic reasons that adult people who are 30 years old experience non-cardiac chest pain.

Anyway, my friend Ryan and I got dressed after twenty-two hours of winter-weather related car accidents, falls, and other injuries. Two hours to go in our shift and we have a chest pain to attend to. We got into the ambulance and started out for this little hamlet that was about three miles from our station. The upscale home we were called to was in a fashionable and expensive gated neighborhood. The house was just inside the main entrance of this sequestered community. It would come to pass that quickly finding his home in a sea of homes would be fortuitous for not only our soon to be patient and his family, but also for Ryan and me.

We got out of the ambulance and the only equipment I was carrying was a blood pressure cuff and a stethoscope. Most of us in EMS know that's about all you need, particularly for the kind of case we were on. We walked up to the door and knocked. Immediately the door opened and there stands a woman around 30 years old with near panic on her face.

She opened the door and immediately refers us to her husband who was sitting on the couch behind her. She said he had been having really bad chest pain since he came home from work at midnight. When she said that, I looked at my wristwatch and noted that it had been more than six hours that he has been suffering with chest pain.

As she continues to talk with Ryan, I begin to check out his vital signs. I made a mental note that his blood pressure was quite elevated, as was his heart rate, and both were considered well outside of the normal range. With my many years of EMS experience, I wouldn't consider these findings unusual. The fact is that just about anything can, and will affect your blood pressure and heart rate. And that certainly includes two strange men in your house with an ambulance parked in your driveway. So, consequently, unless the vital signs are in a near-lethal range, one unusual blood pressure does not a crisis make.

After recording his heart rate and blood pressure, I hear Ryan ask his wife if he is on any kind of prescription medicines or if he has a pre-existing condition. He asks her if he's done anything unusual last night or if he's eaten anything out of the ordinary. What we are both doing was trying to figure out what was happening to rule out a heart problem. What I did instantly notice is that instead of someone being pale and diaphoretic (sweaty) because of a heart problem, this man was as red as a beet and dry to the touch.

Trying to inject what appeared to be a little humor into the conversation, I told him the only thing that was wrong with him was that he was wearing a Dallas Cowboys jacket. I didn't ask the question to put down the Cowboys—or for that matter him as a Cowboy's fan. I did it to see what kind of reaction I would get out of him. Often times you can gauge someone's reaction to a question or a statement you pose to them and instantly know how they are truly feeling.

His reaction was remarkable for having no reaction at all. He just kept sitting on his couch, his arms straight down by his sides, elbows locked with his fists pushing into the couch cushions, and looking down toward the floor. In his case I instinctively knew that he was really in distress and had been for at least six and a half hours. At that moment, I knew (and I think Ryan knew) that this was going to be one of those very rare cases where a young guy without a prior medical history was having the "Big One."

Even though his symptoms weren't classic cardiac symptoms, I couldn't rule out cardiac-type pain or a possible acute myocardial infarction (heart attack). The more I looked at this guy, the more I thought to myself, *Oh man, I think this is the real deal. This poor guy, who had just turned 30 years old, is suffering a heart attack. Holy Christ, Ryan and I had better get things moving.*

Knowing Ryan is one of the finer paramedics there is at Medic 1, I was certain that he was already thinking the same thing. He stayed with him while I went out into the dreadfully cold morning air to retrieve the ambulance cot and oxygen. As is the case with a few houses, you can't get the cot inside without a major fiasco. I didn't want to take a lot of time getting this possibly, and most probably very ill and young man out of his home and into the back of our ambulance. So I brought the oxygen bottle in along with a non-rebreather mask to where the man was still sitting.

As I turned the valve on the portable oxygen bottle and began to immediately fill the plastic reservoir, I watched an expression of growing dread cross his face. Seeing the look of "impending doom" is a huge indicator for those of us in EMS. We've learned over the years that most people instinctively know when they may be approaching their own mortality. Just as I witnessed his change of appearance, I placed the mask over his head and secured it to his face. I told him that we would walk a few steps outside and then down a few more steps to where the ambulance cot awaited him.

Without hesitation, he immediately got up and started walking (yet another sign that this guy believed that he was really in some trouble). As we are walking down the three or four steps and to the cot, Ryan unfolded the blanket and sheet to minimize the cold he was certainly going to feel. To make matters worse, I had to remove his Cowboy's jacket. Now he was bare chested and very cold in the single digit or sub-zero weather. But that's just a matter of superficial comfort. Ryan and I weren't interested in his comfort in that regard and at that particular moment. Remarkably, our patient didn't say a word about the cold or being cold.

As we secured him and the oxygen bottle to the cot, his wife was following us out of their home with a small child in hand. I told her that she shouldn't try to follow us to the hospital because the roads were dangerously snowy and slippery. Since our ambulance was parked next to her car, she could leave whenever she wanted. We loaded our patient into the back of the ambulance and headed to the hospital with the wife in her car prepared to follow.

Suddenly Ryan yelled, "Stine, get back here!" I knew that the patient had either taken a turn for the worse or that our patient was in cardiac arrest. In view of the fact that the ambulance was just crawling as we were backing out, I slammed the gearshift into park and leaped out of the driver's door.

I ran to the back of the ambulance and threw open the right side back door just in time to see our patient go into cardiac arrest. His arms and legs were having contractures, his back was arched, he was redder than he was before (almost purple), and he was exhaling the air from his lungs through tightly pursed lips in a hissing manner. In a strange way, it appeared that the essence of his life was leaving his body.

Ryan is now in a full scramble, turning the power on to our

monitor, retrieving the defibrillator cable, and getting to the patient's chest with defibrillator pads. I quickly reached our and felt for a carotid pulse not expecting to find one. Unfortunately, I was not disappointed. With the patient now without a pulse, and the defibrillator pads not yet in place, I raised my fist and delivered a downward thrust to his chest across the lower third of his sternum. At the time it was the right thing to do because Ryan wasn't ready to deliver the needed electrical shock to his heart.

But, striking a patient's chest with sufficient force to attempt to stimulate the heart into a viable rhythm looks as gruesome as can be. What made things worse, was his wife saw me delivering the "precordial thump" that caused his head to lurch forward and raise off of the cot, and his arms to momentarily flail. I quickly checked for the presence of a carotid pulse and found none. He was still in cardiac arrest.

In a flash Ryan was slapping the two defibrillator pads onto our patient's chest. And just as fast I had the drug box open and a restricting band around his left arm. I was grabbing for an alcohol prep and an IV needle when Ryan was set to defibrillate our patient.

"Don't wait for me! Give me a 3-2-1 countdown and shock him! I'll be out of the way!" I ordered.

As quickly as we were doing things that involved sharp needles, potent medicines, lethal levels of electricity, all in cramped quarters, I can't tell you whether any of it would have passed an OSHA standard or not, but that's what we did. Just as I'm ready to stick him with the needle, Ryan gives me a 3-2-1 countdown in about one second. The moment I got my hands out of the way he delivered the shock.

The patient's heart started beating again, and about as quickly as witnessed by the use of the cardiac monitor, his heart went back into fibrillation. Ryan quickly recharged the defibrillator a second time and shocked him. Again, the heart monitor showed a few complexes complete with pulses with those complexes lasting less than five seconds, and then back into fibrillation.

By this time I had started the IV and secured it heavily to our patient's arm so during this chaotic time it wouldn't accidentally be dislodged from his vein or pulled out of his arm entirely. The moment that was completed, I reached for the drug Lidocaine, an anesthetic that when used intravenously takes the irritability out of the heart muscle and raises the fibrillation threshold.

As I was injecting the drug, Ryan started chest compressions. We had to get that medication circulated and to the heart muscle if our efforts are going to be ultimately successful. As fast as I could push the plunger to the syringe, I gave our patient 100 mg. of Lidocaine. Ryan did another two-dozen compressions and then recharged our life pack defibrillator and delivered another shock.

"No capture on the monitor Cronk, and I don't have a pulse," I yelled to him.

"I know! I know! I can see it too!" he said back to me. "I'm shocking again!"

It took a total of four defibrillations to keep this young man's heart beating. Of course whenever you defibrillate someone and deliver that amount of electrical energy through them, they have a body wide, total body spasm. We were flying around the back end of the ambulance doing many life-saving procedures all in about two minutes.

During these frantic two minutes, the man's wife was watching us from inside her car and witnessing the clinical death and re-suscitation of her husband. As the patient's heart appeared to stabilize, I jumped out of the back of the ambulance to drive to the hospital. That's when I noticed the man's wife just sitting in her car with a terrified look on her face, clutching the steering wheel, and crying her guts out. I don't know if I have ever seen anyone cry harder than she was at that moment. It must have been truly horrific for her.

Since she was only fifteen to twenty feet away, I ran to her car. Seeing that she was extremely distraught and having a white-knuckle grip on the steering wheel, I said to her in a calming and reassuring voice, "Listen to me. Listen to me. Your husband had a cardiac event, but my partner and I have him stabilized. He's going to be all right. Right now I need to know if you will be all right if you're going to try to drive to the hospital. It's really important for you to understand that, and you'll have to pull yourself together as quickly as you can. Do you understand me?"

Still crying and totally unable to talk, she vigorously shook her head, yes. When she shook her head, I continued, "Don't try to follow right behind us, on these icy roads it won't be safe for either of us."

I told her that if we stopped again for her to go around us and continue on to the hospital. Still trembling and shaking like a leaf, she pulled behind us and started to follow us to the hospital. We probably weren't a mile down the road when Ryan shouted to me, "Stine, get back here!" I stopped the ambulance as quickly as possible on the extremely icy road and once again jumped in the back of the ambulance. Ryan had been assessing the patient and his vital signs when he suddenly relapsed into cardiac arrest.

As I quickly gave another bolus of 100mg. of Lidocaine, my partner started chest compressions on our patient and within in a minute the patient was ready for another defibrillation. Ryan delivered at least two more electrical shocks before his heart would beat effectively again. To keep our patient's blood level of Lidocaine therapeutic, I hung a Lidocaine drip and set it for 3mg./min. infusion rate.

I asked whether he wanted to drive and have me stay in the back of our ambulance, or if he was okay with continuing attending to our very critical patient? He assured me he would be okay. I jumped out of the back end of our rig and hustled up to the front, got back behind the wheel, and continued towards the hospital.

Three things I knew: First, that it was as slippery as it ever gets on Michigan roads in the middle of the winter season. Second, our patient was in an extremely unstable, critical condition. And third, Ryan and I were extremely nervous and tense about it. As I eased down the country roads that lead to the city streets and finally to the hospital, I enquired about every two minutes about the condition, vital signs, and cardiac rhythm of our patient. To say the least, things continued to be up and down.

Approximately five minutes subsequent to the last time we stopped the ambulance, our patient went into fibrillation a third time. I asked Ryan if he wanted me to stop and help, but he insisted on just getting to the hospital. While mostly driving—and sometimes sliding—we were able to keep the ambulance between the curbs on the city streets and arrived at the hospital approximately forty-five minutes after we first encountered our patient. We wasted no time in getting him out of the ambulance and into the emergency department where respiratory care and a cardiologist from the cardiovascular lab were all waiting. He survived.

When I think back on that call, it was one that needed to go right. Not because it took uncommon talent to make it an extraordinary save; far from it. It needed to have a successful outcome because so very much in the human condition was at stake. The focal point is the patient who had just turned 30, was suffering a massive, life-threatening heart attack.

Our emergency advanced cardiac life support treatment was in a sense the easy part. The reason is, that if you take this particular patient and treat him in a vacuum, then whether he lives or whether he dies is diminished to the point of "well it's just one person", kind of thought. But we don't live in a vacuum. Most all of us are interdependent in symbiotic relationships. What that means is that if Ryan and I weren't there, or weren't able to save this young man, he would have been missed and other lives would have been changed.

Some of those lives would be changed forever. Parents would have buried a son. A young lady would be a widow, and lastly and perhaps the worst, a young child would never know his or her father.

I can't think of another job where the high stakes of life and death may present itself in a moment's notice. For this reason, the profession of EMS is like no other. When thrust into immediate action, the express result of our efforts in direct patient care and the residual effects on family and friends can last for decades. And if your efforts and labors are successful, you thank God for allowing you to be a part of it.

***

As if the pressure of doing this type of job isn't enough, one thing that makes it all the more intense and pressure packed is when you have a personal investment in that particular call. Many times over the years, I've been called in my professional capacity to help people that I call friends, family, and neighbors.

Other than a few years in the Florida Keys, my parents have pretty much lived here in southwest Michigan their whole lives. Both sets of my grandparents lived the vast majority of their lives here, and are buried locally. With many large multi-generational families in which most members live locally, it's not surprising that I get to know a fair percentage of the people I may run into concerning their need for EMS.

Hundreds of times I've been dispatched to homes to help a neighbor, relative, or friend. When I am scheduled to work at the very same station in which I started in EMS, and if I'm dispatched for a medical emergency to a private residence, then there's one chance in three that I'll know the person or at least be acquainted with their family.

One day while on duty, my partner Anthony Pantaleo and I had just completed a very forgettable call for a sick old lady in one of the nursing homes. As we are getting back to the Bridgman/ Baroda and Lake Township area, we decided to stop at a little mom-and-pop diner owned by Dan and Jayne Daniel. (Dan is a paramedic for Medic 1, as well as a volunteer for the township fire department.)

Dan always carried at least one or two hand-held radio/pager units with him at all times; today was no different. While Anthony and I were in the restaurant, the whole restaurant heard his pager being activated by the local county sheriff's dispatch. We heard that the Lake Township Fire Department was being called to come to the aid of someone not breathing. At first, I was irritated that we weren't called first, yet we listened to the dispatch.

Dan asked us if we heard the call. We did and headed out behind Dan who was in his private vehicle. He told us that the incident was on Snow Road between Gast and California Roads. I had family in that area and held my breath that we weren't headed to one of their homes.

I was relieved when we passed by my relatives' house, but we pulled into the driveway of a house that was owned by my dad's friend, Irv Poschke. Irv and his wife Margaret had been life-long residents of our small town, and Irv had just retired from the local school district. He was one of the nicest men I knew. He always greeted others with a smile, a kind word, and a handshake. He was the accordion player in a Polka band that my Dad had put together back in the mid 1960's. I spent many hours listening to them practice and play at local wedding receptions, various social parties like the Fireman's Ball, Hunter's Ball, and New Year's Eve events.

A minute or two prior to our arrival, we heard that the local police and the fire department medical first responder's were doing CPR. As we wheeled into the Poschke's driveway, I remember thinking, "Oh shit, this is Irv and Margaret's house!" I jumped out of the ambulance, threw open the side door of the ambulance, grabbed our airway box, and dashed into the house.

Lying supine on the floor was a guy that I didn't recognize. As I'm briskly walking toward the men doing CPR, I looked at Margaret who was sitting on the couch crying and shaking uncontrollably. I said, "Margaret, I'm Jim Stine. Is this Irv? Is this Irv?"

"Yes! Yes!" she blurts out. I couldn't believe it. It didn't look anything like him. He was totally lifeless and his face was a very deep purple in color. I thought, "Oh man, Irv is dead for sure. There's just no way he's ever going to make it."

Together, along with the police and fire personnel, we joined the firefighters already doing CPR and started to do our advanced life support work. The firemen had just defibrillated him once without success. I quickly told those at Irv's side that they were doing a good job with CPR, and not to stop until we were able to assess his heart rhythm. Other firefighters and police officers retrieved equipment from the ambulance, and still others were moving furniture to create an adequate working space for the rescuers.

Just as importantly, another firefighter was explaining to Margaret what was happening in the course of our life-saving efforts. He made sure she understood that we were doing the necessary things that were needed if Irv was going to have any chance of survival. The firefighter explained to Margaret that we weren't wasting any time, and that we weren't doing any unnecessary procedures. I can only imagine what it must be like for a loved one to sit idle while their way of life is disintegrating before their eyes.

As Anthony, Dan, and I knelt next to Irv, Anthony intubated Irv and then handed the ventilating duties over to one of the firemen. Dan switched the defibrillator pads from the firefighters AED to our Lifepack 12 monitor and then placed the four limb leads on the corners of Irv's chest and abdomen. Now for the first time we would be able to see what kind of heart rhythm Irv's heart would be showing us.

Meanwhile, I looked for a reliable vein on Irv's right arm and couldn't find one. Anthony immediately states, "Jim, I think I can get an E-J". (An E-J is the external jugular vein that is on the side of a persons' neck.)

I promptly handed Anthony a 16-gauge quick-cath IV catheter and prepared a 1000ml. IV bag of normal saline for drug administration. Anthony inserted the catheter into Irv's neck and after I attached the IV line to the end of the catheter he heavily taped it in place. We now had a good route into Irv's cardiovascular system to get definitive drug therapy underway.

In less than three minutes, all of the different rescuers and levels of EMS came together and had started CPR, cleared a work area, placed the AED machine on Irv, defibrillated him once, hauled in arm loads of emergency medical equipment, put the cardiac monitor leads on his chest, inserted an advanced airway, delivered high flow oxygen, secured an IV, and had started drug therapy.

With the way Irv looked I didn't expect much more than asystole, which would indicate no cardiac activity, and would be seen on our cardiac monitor as a flat line and likely mean irreversible death. What I saw was a fine ventricular fibrillation (V-fib). It's not great but it's better than asystole and at least we could work with it. I immediately injected into Irv's IV line 1mg. of Epinephrine and 1mg. of Atropine. After a minute or two of really vigorous CPR, we defibrillated Irv for the second time into a type of rhythm that we call PEA or Pulseless Electrical Activity.

Simply stated, that's when you have a regular and recognizable heart rhythm that you can see on your cardiac monitor, but your patient doesn't have a corresponding pulse. That's bad. When PEA is observed it's an indication that although the heart muscle is willing, it is unable to generate a life-sustaining pulse and blood pressure.

After seeing the heart rhythm PEA, CPR was resumed and I gave Irv another bolus of epinephrine. After perhaps only thirty seconds of additional CPR we were able to find a pulse. Unfortunately, after only ten to fifteen seconds of a pulsed heart rhythm, Irv's heart slipped back into ventricular fibrillation. The Lake Township firefighters quickly restarted their vigorous chest compressions and I gave our patient a bolus of 100mg. of the drug, Lidocaine.

As I was infusing the Lidocaine, Dan quickly recharged the defibrillator, and within 20 seconds he delivered 300 joules of electrical energy through Irv's chest. No result.

"Recharge and hit him again! " I told Dan. Ten seconds later Dan shocked him again. This time Irv's heart jumped into yet another rhythm called ventricular tachycardia (V-tach). It's not as bad as the heart just "quivering", but it's not life sustaining either.

"Anthony, does he have a pulse with that?"

"I can't feel one Jim."

"Dan, we need to cardiovert right now. Hit the synchronizer button and let's shock him again!" I said.

The difference between defibrillation and cardioversion is that with defibrillation the electrical energy is delivered the instant you hit the fire button. With cardioversion, you want to synchronize exactly when that same energy is delivered. It's vital to give that shock precisely at the right moment in time during a single heartbeat. Resuscitation efforts require it if your patient has any kind of regular heart rhythm.

Without hesitation, Dan again recharged the defibrillator, activated the synchronizer, and again hit Irv with 300 joules of electrical energy. Irv's heart responded by showing us a normal sinus rhythm. As soon as I saw that beautiful sinus rhythm I was soon informed that we did indeed have a pulse that we saw on our cardiac monitor.

With that information, I started another IV on Irv and hung

a Lidocaine drip, which means I gave Irv a continuous dose of Lidocaine so his heart would hopefully not slip back into fibrillation. By this time, the firefighters who weren't doing CPR had retrieved the cot and a backboard from our ambulance. They were just waiting for the word to put Irv on the board and place him on the cot.

As soon as I had secured the additional IV, I said to the firefighters, "Okay guys, let's move him right now before anything else happens!" They sprang into action to get Irv on to the backboard and place and secure him to our ambulance stretcher.

They were removing Irv from his home and Anthony, Dan, and I were busy gathering the needed equipment to put back into the ambulance to continue the vital and critical care that we were administering. Still others were busy cleaning up the mess that is always left behind during such a rescue effort. Each time there seems to be a big sack full of trash and disposable medical supplies that are left all over the area when efforts such as this are concluded.

I followed the firefighters who were wheeling the cot that contained this close and personal friend, and quickly climbed into the patient compartment from the side door. As they hoisted the cot and rolled it into place, I hastily grabbed the Ambu-bag and resumed Irv's rescue breathing as they hoisted the cot and rolled it into place. Without delay Anthony and Dan joined me in the back of the ambulance to reconnect oxygen lines, cardiac cables, a blood pressure monitor, pulse-ox and carbon dioxide monitors, re-hang multiple IV bags, and to help me reassess Irv's condition...or as we say, to get things "squared away".

Even though as a paramedic you attempt to get things squared away, the fact of the matter is that when a person is just resuscitated from the jaws of death, things are generally far from being stable or squared away. With those types of situations, we try and have very little trouble in getting an MFR, police officer, or firefighter to drive the ambulance to the hospital. This is done so both of the paramedics or professional ambulance crew members can be in the patient compartment with this type of very critical patient.

Everyone concerned—and especially our patient, was very

fortunate to have yet another paramedic to lend a hand in the manner of an MFR. With Anthony behind the steering wheel, Dan offered to assist me with Irv's emergency cardiac care. Knowing that in the short term Irv's successful resuscitation was still in question, I accepted Dan's offer. As we got under way to the hospital I felt that we would be fortunate to deliver a live patient. As far as the thought of quality of life was concerned, I had little doubt that Irv's family would ever be the same.

About seven minutes into our twenty-minute trip to the nearest hospital, Irv again went into cardiac arrest. He slipped from a normal heart rhythm (normal sinus rhythm) into ventricular fibrillation. Dan, without delay, started CPR as I got another dose of Lidocaine ready to administer. I injected another 75mg. of Lidocaine and upped the dose of continued Lidocaine. Dan continued vigorous CPR for another thirty to forty seconds. Two defibrillations later Irv's heartbeat was here to stay.

We sped to the hospital; things really started to look favorable. Within five minutes after the seventh and last defibrillation, Irv started to breathe on his own. At first it was just a breath every twenty seconds or so. Soon it was a breath every six to eight seconds along with a little hand movement. I have witnessed this type of reaction many times during vigorous resuscitation efforts, with young or middle-aged relatively healthy people.

I was simply astonished. To think perhaps Irv may have a chance at survival at all was surprising. At the time I was thinking that just surviving was all anyone could reasonably expect, considering the shape he was in at his home just thirty minutes prior.

A few days later, I saw Irv's wife Margaret, and their son Jim walk in through the emergency room entrance to make a visit to the coronary care unit. They were quick to tell me that Irv was awake but not quite "with it" just yet. I could tell that they were truly hopeful that he would make a full recovery. Frankly speaking, I really had my doubts. I couldn't see how someone who was purple in color, pulseless with dilated and fixed pupils, would ever make a "full recovery". In the real, non-Hollywood world, that just doesn't happen.

I heard a couple of weeks later that he had been discharged

to go home a week or two after his near life-ending event. At first I thought that Margaret just wanted him home, to make him comfortable, and to get him around familiar surroundings. I had all of these images in my mind of Margaret feeding him, helping him dress himself, and to simply do the normal daily things that we all do (and for the most part just take for granted). I really thought that for the Poschke family, that was going to be the best possible outcome. I've never been so delighted to be wrong.

A couple of months after his discharge I happened to be driving past his house. There he was, sitting atop his riding lawn mower zipping around his yard. At that moment, I'd never been so proud of all the people who came together to help a friend during the most critical and darkest hour of his life. I would be less than truthful if I didn't admit to walking just a little taller. Mostly, I felt extraordinarily proud of my profession and all of the great people who make it what it is today.

***

August 7, 2008, is a day that I'll never forget. I was on duty and due to our shift rotation I was assigned to our Lake Township station, which is conveniently just a little more than a half mile from my home. At the time I was working with a 24-year-old named Brian Patterson.

We were doing what we call "sitting point"; sitting between two coverage areas. Our ambulance would sit at a point somewhere in between the two zones in order to have coverage in both areas. A call came in that a motorcycle versus car personal injury (P.I.) accident had occurred at the corner of Linco Road and Red Arrow Highway. Red Arrow is a four-lane highway, and Linco is a small two-way road that Ts into the highway. Because of the mechanism of potential injuries involving anything from minor "road rash" to a fatality are great, it's an emergency response for sure.

Brian flipped the emergency lights on and roared off to that destination that was about five minutes away. We were about halfway there when our dispatch center contacted us and stated that the county police were on the scene, the driver of the motor-

97

cycle was in bad shape, and for us to "step on it!" We were already clipping along at a fairly high rate of speed when I told Brian that no matter what anybody (including myself) says, he should never go any faster than what he feels comfortable with, no matter the circumstances.

As we approached the scene, it became apparent that there were more than the usual amount of people and cars we would normally expect to see. There is a small commercial building right at the corner of this particular intersection that is the local home of the American Cancer Society. On this day, they happened to be conducting some sort or rummage or yard sale to raise funds. There were cars parked in their small parking lot and along Red Arrow Highway.

From what I understand, the driver of the car couldn't see the oncoming traffic and pulled out on to the highway and into the motorcycle's right of way. I found out later that the impact point was just behind the driver's left, front wheel.

Brian stopped the ambulance maybe twenty feet from where our patient was lying. I then saw a good friend of mine and former Benton Township police officer, Kim Fowler. He was holding the helmeted head of the victim who was lying in a prone position in the middle of the paved four-lane highway. When I jumped out of the ambulance, and took a few brisk strides toward the victim, the other bystanders quickly parted so I could move unencumbered. As I looked at Kim, he looked back at me with a very dire look on his face. At that same moment I saw the victim, that would in a matter of a few short seconds become (for me) the most important patient that I've had in a long, long time.

I saw the prone body of a man who was husky, and had been riding a motorcycle while wearing a T-shirt that read: Lake Township Fire and Rescue. It was my good friend Dan from Medic 1, one who assisted in the successful resuscitation of Irv. At that same moment, Kim Fowler says to me, "Jim, its Dan!"

Now things and thoughts are happening in milliseconds. As I'm still about ten feet from his side, in an instant I answered Kim, "I see that!"

In that same instant, I thought that maybe Dan had perhaps

sustained some "road rash" and maybe a broken leg, or he would be complaining about some general back pain, or something simple. I thought that Kim was holding his head as a way of telling Dan to just to be still, and wait for one of his colleagues to show up.

During the next few milliseconds, I said to Kim, "How is he? Is he awake?" Before Kim could tell me no, and as I took another stride, I could hear Dan breathing. He had what we call deep "snoring respirations", and I knew that when I examined him he would be comatose.

Snoring respirations are a bad neurological sign that is highly indicative of a severe head injury. As I quickly knelt next to Dan's head and shoulders, I put the side of my face right on the pavement and pried his eyes open. Dan's eyes had rolled toward the back of his head and both were pointing in the two o'clock position; known as a disconjugate gaze. Over the years I'd seen many dozens of these types of head injuries associated with high velocity blunt force trauma, gunshot wounds, and falls from bone breaking heights. It's been my experience that over half of them have resulted in fatalities.

Brian and I had to do everything right. There would be no wasted movements and efficiency would be at a premium. The other firefighters on scene too were friends with Dan and would have to stay calm. No matter what we did or how well we did it, that sick feeling in the pit of my stomach told me that my good friend just might die this very day.

Just that fast, I felt anger (at the situation), highly confident in what we all had to accomplish in a few minutes, and more than a little scared that all of this might not go quite right. If he survived his trip to the hospital, he would need the best efforts of the many doctors, nurses, and technicians awaiting his arrival in the emergency room. He needed the best that I could give him.

As I snapped up from looking into his eyes, I said to my partner and the firefighters, "Brian, get a backboard, you (one of the firemen) get the towel roles, and you (another fireman) get the cot! I'll get a collar! Kim, hold his head and don't move!"

I had everybody running for this and that while thinking, "Oh my

God, I can't believe this is happening." Within a matter of seconds, I was back at Dan's side. It was impossible to apply the cervical collar while his helmet was still on, and we couldn't safely remove it while he was lying face down. I decided that his helmet would have to come off and that it would be better if we did it when we placed Dan in a supine position.

I then took over the management of Dan's head and neck, and I had Kim move to Dan's torso in order to help my partner and the firemen get Dan rolled to a supine position, and onto our backboard. We were all very careful to align and keep Dan's spine in a normal anatomical position. Once we got him on his back, I could see that the chinstrap appeared unusually tight to the point that it may be slightly choking him, and that his tongue looked as though it was swelling and protruding from his mouth.

I called for trauma shears, still not believing that I was working on one of my closest and dearest friends. Within twenty seconds I had Dan's helmet removed from his head and a "Stiff-Neck" cervical collar applied around his neck. The placement of the much-needed collar was also a little tricky because Dan was one of those guys who was so stocky that he didn't appear to have much of a neck. My partner and the firefighters were applying the restraining backboard straps around Dan's body. In just a few seconds we had fully secured our friend and colleague to a backboard, placed it on a cot, and hustled him to our ambulance.

Since there were several members of the rescue team around our cot, I ran ahead of it and jumped into the ambulance to start the process of more definitive care. I immediately turned on our main oxygen tank and cardiac monitor, pulled our drug and IV bag from its cabinet, and opened our advanced airway box. By now Dan was being slid into the back of our ambulance.

Brian, without delay, climbed in behind the cot, looked at me with just a little bit of dread in his eyes, and said, "What do you want me to do?"

Seeing that Brian's stress level might be "red-lining" I said, "Do you think you can start an IV? If you can do that, that's what I need from you. Hang a bag and run it at a 'keep open rate' for now!"

"You got it!"

I wrapped our automatic blood pressure cuff around his arm and slapped electrodes to his chest so we could better assess his cardiovascular system. I was thinking almost out loud, "Please Brian, just get that IV. I have to get Dan intubated before he throws-up all over and aspirates."

After getting Dan off of the pavement, protecting his airway was my next worry. I knew that most people that have sustained a head injury of this magnitude almost always vomit. If you don't have their airway secure you may run the risk of a highly-compromised airway, and a patient whose survival is now much less possible. Dan didn't need anything compromising an already questionable outcome to his very survival.

I was contemplating whether to attempt a regular oral intubation or try the nasal route. Since Dan had a neck that started at his ear lobes and ended at his shoulders, and I already had a stiff neck cervical collar in place. The last thing I wanted to do was to manipulate his neck to any degree. I decided to secure his airway by putting an endotracheal tube up through his nose and down into his trachea.

I have intubated people in that fashion many times in the past and always due to very traumatic injuries. What I've learned is that sometimes it is difficult, and once in a while there are complications. Sometimes, if there is considerable facial trauma (like broken facial and nasal bones) it may be impossible to push the tube up the nose and down into the trachea.

Other times, such a maneuver will cause a nose bleed that may be quite severe, and you get blood pouring down the back of the throat as well. To top it all off, if you don't time the insertion just right, the tube will wind up in the esophagus. If you don't push it down far enough, the end of the tube will be in the back of the throat and my attempt to secure airway will have failed.

The 6mm tube that I inserted correctly into Dan's trachea went down very easily and it was probably (and gladly) one of the easiest nasal intubations that I have ever done. I was immensely relieved when I could tell that Dan was now breathing through the tube. As it turned out, there wasn't much time to waste, because about ninety seconds after his airway was secured, he did in fact vomit. Now instead of being in a panic about a highly compromised airway, I wasn't concerned about it at all.

While all of this is going on, I yelled out to Kim and asked him if he could drive the ambulance to the hospital, while my partner Brian and I tended to Dan. Without any hesitation, Kim jumped behind the wheel and said, "Jim, just let me know when you're ready to go."

We quickly recorded Dan's blood pressure and I said, "Let's go Kim, and don't spare the horses!"

As we are traveling through traffic on our way to the hospital, Brian started the IV that I needed. I fastened an oxygen hose to the end of the endotracheal tube that I had just inserted by cutting the end off of a nasal cannula, and taping the open end to the end of the endotracheal tube. I then evacuated Dan's mouth from the emesis that had been laying there for the last couple of minutes.

Once his airway was fully secure, and with the administration of oxygen, I could take a brief minute to reassess Dan's injuries and his neurological condition. That was the first time that I noticed that Dan's left leg and foot were abducted (flopped over toward the outside of his body) and I thought for sure that he probably had a fractured left hip or possibly pelvic fractures. But I was so preoccupied with his head injury I didn't even mention it to the nurse when I called the emergency room staff to advise them of the patient they would be receiving.

I didn't expect any positive change in his coma status, and sadly there wasn't. There have been countless times over my years in EMS, that I have seen victims of head injuries who were exhibiting the same symptoms that my friend and colleague was showing; many of them having died. To the best of my knowledge, not very many have returned to any semblance of a normal life that they may have had prior to their accident. From what I was told by the attending emergency room physician, the type of brain injury that Dan suffered made his chances for recovery between 5-10%. I was disheartened, and I felt so helpless that I didn't know what to do or say to anyone.

Dan's wife Jayne, who ran the family diner, was one of the nicest and kindest people I have ever met. Outside of her diner, she was active in the Lake Charter Township Firefighters Women's Auxiliary, and was always in the forefront of financial, moral, and community support when misfortune strikes a member or family of our small community. Dan often told me that through their twenty-five plus years of marriage they were yet to have their first real argument let, alone verbal fight.

I know that's hard to believe, but if you ever saw the two of them together you would be hard pressed to find another couple who were so happy, contented, and at ease with each other. He always treated her like it was their first date. She responded to him with unconditional love, affection, and support. So seeing her at the hospital broke my heart.

Jayne and her sister Cheryl, walked through the same entrance in which we had brought Dan about twenty minutes earlier. At the time I was struggling with the paperwork and needed to take an emotional and mental break from the words I was writing. I was documenting devastating head injuries that may kill, or at the least leave lifelong and lasting injuries to a loved and cherished friend. I got up from the desk where I was seated and walked into Trauma room #1 where Dan was being assessed and treated. He was being cared for by Dr. Walker, probably one of the most competent, ex-perienced, and talented emergency room physician's that I have ever worked with.

As I was coming out of the emergency room and back into the ambulance entrance area, Jayne and I saw each other. She had the most terrified look I ever witnessed. Her expression was one of paralyzing fear and trepidation. Barely above a whisper she said to me, "How is he Jim?"

I said, "I don't know. It doesn't look good."

At that time we embraced and she cried so hard on my shoulder that she made me cry. God, I felt so bad for her. As the emergency room staff further stabilized Dan, they rushed him to the X-ray de-partment for an emergency CT scan.

During that time, there were no less than twenty co-workers from Medic 1, both off-duty as well as on-duty personnel who came to the emergency room when they had heard of what had happened. By this time, Jayne had been sequestered into a small private room that is used to hold family members in a place where the attending physician can talk to them privately. It's a place where bad news is usually given to family members by the medical doctors on staff, and a place where family members can console each other when the news that a loved one has passed away or is so ill or injured that their survival is in doubt.

Soon after, Dan's current road partner and long-time friend Ray came into the emergency room. He looked so grim and serious that his face looked gray. He came up to me and softly said, "I heard that you were the one that brought Dan in."

"Yeah, I brought him in about thirty minutes ago."

"Well thank God for that. I'm really glad you were the one there for Dan," he replied. It was a nice thing for Ray to say, and I deeply appreciated his confidence in my treatment. But at the time I felt about as helpless as the captain of the Titanic.

"What do you think, Jim?"

I shrugged my shoulders and simply said, "Ray, I think that Dan just might die today." Even as I said that to him, I couldn't believe what I was saying. It seemed so surreal.

Over the next forty-five minutes most of the people from Medic 1, the hospital staff, and Dan's many friends and relatives, rushed to the hospital to inquire on his condition and to be with Jayne. Several of them thanked Brian and me for our efforts in Dan's pre-hospital emergency care. It was all quite nice, but if there was ever a call that I didn't need to be thanked for, it was that one.

I felt so terrible and so disheartened that it was one of those extremely rare times that I wished that I didn't know anything about anatomy, physiology, closed-head injuries, EMS, or any of it. It was one of those times that I thought for sure that ignorance was bliss. But none of that would change what was.

Within ten minutes after we had arrived at the hospital with Dan, Bronson Methodist Hospital in Kalamazoo was called, and an emergency request for their helicopter was issued. It's a sixty-mile trip by interstate highway; by air it's only a matter of maybe fifteen to twenty minutes. The helicopter touched down at our local hospital and their highly specialized team was inside reassessing and getting Dan ready for his airlift to Bronson, the regional level-one trauma center in southwest Michigan.

We later learned that Dan had suffered shearing injuries to his brain that caused many micro-bleeds. What I thought was a hip or maybe a pelvic fracture, actually turned out to be an eight-inch separation in his pelvis with a sacral fracture. The fractures and pelvic separations caused a lot of blood loss but surgery was out of the question due to his head injury. Later after Dan's head injury had stabilized, he went through successful pelvic surgery.

About three weeks after the accident, he returned by ambulance to our local hospital to undergo physical, occupational, and neurological rehabilitation for many months. A prominent doctor of neuropsychology told me that the very earliest a cognitive assessment can be done to ascertain Dan's long-term abilities was a minimum of six months. He said it usually takes up to two years to fully assess and understand just where Dan's mental status would be. His memory both long-term and short-term, his emotional state, cognition, sensory and motor function, physical, and occupational abilities are in question and may not fully be answered for several years.

Dan had a volunteer and professional career in EMS that spanned more than forty years. His service as a firefighter with the Lake Charter Township Fire Department lasted more than twenty-five years. He nobly and honorably served his country during the Vietnam conflict; performing duties as a firefighter on a military base near Saigon, South Vietnam. His selfless and altruistic demeanor exemplified what one person can do to make a difference in any community.

More than 700 people waited in a line more than 100-yards long for two hours to participate in a spaghetti dinner benefit in his honor. Weeks later, hundreds showed up for a day-long hog roast. Approximately three weeks later more than 150 cyclists paid tribute to Dan during a motorcycle ride; all to let a valued friend, neighbor, and colleague know that in his time of need the whole community was there to support him just as he had always been there for them in their darkest and most troubled hour of need.

As for me, the only thing I know for sure, is that my life is much richer with him in it. I love you, Dan. Best of luck.

Chapter 6
PUPPIES IN THE WORKPLACE

Since I started my EMS career, things in the workplace have changed. I vividly remember at the tender age of 19, working at my aunt and uncle's plastic injection mold factory and contemplating just the possibility of a career in EMS. That was in the early months of 1977 while I was going through the basic EMT course at our local community college. It was the first time an EMS course was being taught locally, and not knowing whether or if another EMT course would be offered for a second time, I wiggled my way into the class.

I knew at the time that the local township volunteer ambulance service was having difficulty staffing a reliable crew. I also knew that I was the only person who currently resided within the township who was going to have an EMT certificate (there was no state EMT licensure at that time) once I had successfully completed the five-month course in May of that year.

My dad's younger brothers Mike and Russ, were volunteer firemen who often responded to ambulance calls. I asked them about my chances of getting a job locally rather than going to Benton Harbor. At the time, I wasn't interested in being involved in the ambulance wars currently being waged between two private companies that were running on a shoestring budget. Rampart and Action ambulances were two services that didn't have reliable pay days or work schedules.

I remember being told at the time of how one group of guys from one of the ambulance companies would vandalize their rival's ambulance. Then I would hear about the obligatory retaliation. Once, both ambulance companies responded to the same car accident in which the driver of a car was injured. As the first crew arrived on the scene and was attending to the injured patient, the crew of the competing ambulance service arrived on the scene, removed the cot from their competitor's ambulance, and kicked it down a steep embankment, essentially "stealing" the patient from the first crew. This type of thing was rather commonplace.

I wanted no part of it. I was a kid who, with a little luck, would get to run emergency ambulance calls in his own hometown. After talking with my uncle Mike, he told me that I should go and see a man named Ron Germain who would point me in the right direction. Ron was the Lake Township treasurer and a volunteer firefighter. Like both of my uncles, he also ran a fair amount of ambulance calls. So on a Saturday afternoon, I went to Ron's house and told him that I was looking for a job to run ambulance calls during those hours that the township was finding difficult to fill.

He was very receptive to the idea of having someone run calls during the daytime hours, but I needed to talk with the supervisor of the township. After I told him that I had just obtained my EMT certification, he asked my salary request. I told him I could do it for the tidy sum of $8,500 a year. Although he didn't say anything outright, I got the very distinct impression that he was happy with my answer. We talked briefly about what he thought would be expected of me if I were hired. As we talked, I got the feeling that I was just what they were looking for, and left to go see the township supervisor.

After I arrived at the home of the township supervisor, I told him the same story that I had just told to the township treasurer. He told me to come to the next board meeting, which was just a few short days away. After that particular board meeting, I had a job running ambulance calls in my own hometown, and was an automatic member of the Lake Township Fire Department. Life was looking great, and at that moment I knew it would be my life's calling.

By this time, the two private ambulance companies in Benton Harbor folded. As a result, several local communities formed a multi-jurisdictional, municipally-owned ambulance company called Medic 1, which I joined on August 1, 1979.

I quickly realized, that the guys I would be working with were carbon copies of me. These pirates would sacrifice a virgin and a week's pay to run a high-velocity trauma or a bad shooting. For the most part, they did it for the thrill (better known as an adrenaline rush) of the job. Like me, they wanted to be able to do something that meant more than stamping out widgets or pushing a pencil around for eight hours a day. Most people think that saving a life is the ultimate thing that one human being can do for another. That may be so, and it is gratifying, but it's also much more than that.

The number of times I have been called to actually restore the life to someone in cardiac arrest, that has not only a high degree of survivability but also of viability, is relatively small. Most of the time, the call is to help someone who has either chest pain, shortness of breath, has been in a motor vehicle accident, has hurt themselves from a fall, suffered an allergic reaction to prescription drugs or bee stings, or numerous other serious non-life threatening events.

For me, it was—and still is, the dedication of the high stakes responsibility of the emergency call itself. To have the responsibility in my hands that I would be called to save or greatly alter a life on a somewhat regular basis, is still awe-inspiring. After responding to my first ambulance call decades ago, I still enjoy the thrill, excitement, and ultimately the immense satisfaction of battling mortality and morbidity. It is singularly what makes EMS unlike any other profession in the world.

Speaking of the dedication to the profession, more than twenty-five years ago, then executive director Bill Gebhard, put out a company-wide directive that stated ambulance crews (if they wanted to continue their employment) would all have to become licensed paramedics. He gave those who were just EMT's (and that was everybody except the five of us) a year or two, to achieve the above stated level of licensure.

The vast majority of those EMT's, who were my colleagues at that time, took up that challenge and became, for the most part very good and even great paramedics. It was also stated that we wouldn't hire or place on the ambulance anyone who wasn't a paramedic and who didn't have several years of experience.

Oh, those were the days. It's just a shame that the general public didn't know just how talented, educated, experienced, and dedicated their public servants who staffed their emergency ambulances were at that time. Today, as I punch the time clock to start my shift, I look across the large room and I find myself drawing some comparisons, contrasts, and conclusions.

The first is, that when I first started at Medic 1, for years there was virtually no turnover. There were part-time people who literally waited years for a full-time spot. As some of the guys who were here at Medic 1 when I started retired out, they seemed to be replaced with people who didn't have the same zest and dedication as the people who were my contemporaries. I hear way too much complaining about "who's up for the next call," and complaining about working too many hours and not getting enough sleep, and on, and on. The fact is, that there is always going to be another call to respond to, the hours are long, and consequently there are times where sleep is in short supply. You've got to understand that going into the business... so man-up and get over it!

I vividly remember being in my mid-20s and running calls all day and all night, and not thinking a thing of it. It was just they way it was. On top of that, as much as some political people talk about the value of life, none of us were getting rich running ambulance calls. My conclusion is that for the most part, the type of dedication and toughness that was commonplace for more than twenty years, is for the most part, absent. Because of that palpable lack of dedication and toughness, there has been a large turnover here at Medic 1. The fact is, that in the last two years I've seen more people leave Medic 1 than I did the first dozen years I worked here.

The second comparison, contrast, and conclusion is the number of women in EMS today. When I started my first job running ambulance calls with the Lake Township Fire Department, there were zero women on the department, and therefore zero women operating on the ambulance. A little more than two years later after starting at Medic 1, there was just one woman who was a regular, full-time street medic. Today at Medic 1, the current tally is a ratio of 3:1 for men to women.

It took me a long time to be convinced that women in general would fit in to this business. My biggest concern was with safety and security. Let's face it, 99% of the time two men are going to have less of a problem than one man and one woman—or worse yet, two women, in the event of some sort of a physical confrontation.

National statistics will show that EMS providers are in a business that ranks very high in deadly assaults. As for me, I've been on the wrong end of an assault with a gun once, and a knife twice. That's not to mention that since beginning my career in EMS, I've never been in more fist fights and wrestling matches since I was a young kid in grade school.

My second thought, was whether the constant lifting and carrying of patients, ambulance cots, and equipment would present acute as well as chronic injuries, and so forth. Although there have been injuries that some of the ladies have suffered from their professional duties, they don't seem to be any more prone to acute injury than their male counterparts.

Lastly, I have to admit that I thought about the "sexual" component. Is there, or has there been sex on the job at Medic 1? Yes, and plenty of it. Is anybody going to admit it? Not a chance. But, believe me, there has been loads of it. Is it unlike any other work place in this country where men and women are working side by side in close quarters? Probably not. So, as far as I'm concerned, it's a non-issue.

The third comparison, contrast, and conclusion that I see are on display at our central station. I see it when I'm on duty. I see all too often paramedics who have had less than six months of experience who are working with basic EMT's. Several years ago that would have been unconscionable. Now, according to the current management, it's "good enough". After all, "they have a license".

On the job and away from the job I see and interact with several members of law enforcement. They often ask me what's up with some of the ambulance personnel? They have noticed that many of the crews don't appear to have a real good grasp on what's going on with the calls. They've told me that the "new people" don't appear to be very confident in what to do in some of the pressure situations.

For me, this kind of commentary comes as no surprise. That type of comment would not have been uttered by anyone in law enforcement fifteen or more years ago. The inevitable conclusion is that the overall talent at all levels of EMS and its management (presently at Medic 1), is just not there.

Another comparison and conclusion I see, is when I listen to what some of these "new experts" have to say, and how they know this, or are sure of that. Sometimes, I just shake my head and have to laugh to myself. It's obvious to me that some of these "new" paramedics don't even realize that they don't know what they don't know.

A few of these brand new paramedics who are working with their first license, in which the ink has yet to dry, think the same thing that the current management thinks. They think that just because they possess a license they are every bit as able and qualified to do the things veteran guys have been doing for years. The reality of the situation is that this kind of thinking is really dangerous because serious mistakes in patient care are going to happen.

Some of the veteran guys at Medic say that in order to even have an opinion (let alone think that you have all of the answers) on EMS operations or in EMS in general, you should have to work as a street medic for at least five years. That's about right.

As I look back and remember my early days, I thought that I could save the planet. I also didn't know that I didn't know. It didn't take long at all to get slapped in the face with a strong dose of reality. In that respect, the new paramedics are just like a few of us veterans; we've all made mistakes. Most of us will admit that we've made bad mistakes, and I've chronicled a few of my own.

The difference is, that when I started my employment at Medic 1, there were no mentors, no veteran paramedics to "show you the ropes"; and no other highly-trained medical personnel to guide and watch over you and the well being of the patient. There was only a voice on the other end of the radio-telemetry that was supposed to be a doctor, but was almost always a nurse; neither of which had a thought of what you were trying to deal with, and not an inkling of an idea of the working conditions in which you were trying to do it in.

Sometimes, because of mechanical malfunction or "dead spots" in radio transmission areas, you didn't even have that voice to lean on. When I first started at Medic 1, I didn't even have the token luxury of having a partner who was a paramedic. When push came to shove, if I didn't do it, it didn't get done. If I screwed up (and I did), the patient would be the one to suffer for it. Being not quite 22 years old and taking on all of this responsibility for your patient, the account-ability to the medical director whose license you're working under, and the liability of all of it if you screwed up, became at times almost unbearable.

About two years after I joined Medic I, a guy by the name of Dave Ingeson came to work there. As far as raw intelligence is concerned, he was probably one of the smartest men to ever grace the threshold of our ambulance company. When he got his job here, he had just completed his paramedic training. To this day, he still is the only person to get a job here without first working as a basic EMT. The fact was that Dave never worked on any ambulance before he came to Medic.

The only reason he was chosen by management was to fill out the spot next to me that was currently being filled by a basic EMT. Anyway, he had zero experience. Perhaps management thought that at least he was a paramedic and that any paramedic would be better than a well-seasoned basic EMT. If that was the case, then from my point of view, it is skewed thinking. In fact, 100% of the time, I will take a really good EMT over a lousy paramedic or one who has zero experience any day.

Nonetheless, he was there and I knew immediately that at least he had the mental capacity to learn how to put into action what he had learned in the classroom. Another side to this business is the emotional toughness that is needed. Dave had no problem whatsoever with that either. He still is one of the calmest and most collected people I've ever seen work in EMS. However, his first day on the job was very telling in why having a paramedic license is not "good enough."

His first day on the job was with me. By this time I had been working with a really good basic EMT by the name of Dave Hawkins for almost eighteen months, and had pretty much gotten my act together. So, now I felt fairly comfortable with having to work with the "new guy." After some small talk, I gave Dave a tour of the inside of the ambulance and then a tour of the two main hospitals in which we took nearly all of our patients.

Our first call together was for a house fire in a neighborhood not far from our station. The call Dave and I received was for the possibility that there was an elderly female trapped in the blaze. They were right. By the time the firefighters got to her she was little more than a skeleton. So in fact, his first call was functionally no call at all. His next call would be totally different.

As Dave and I were sitting idly by at the old dilapidated fire station, in which we were housed just waiting for some poor soul to have a personal disaster, the phone rang. Our dispatcher yelled out to us that there was a stabbing at the local high school parking lot. Instantly we leaped out of our chairs, slid down the fire pole, jumped into our ambulance, and roared off.

The high school was only about seven city blocks away and by the time we funneled through the traffic both vehicular and pedestrian, we found a 17-year-old female student lying supine and lifeless on the blacktop parking lot. There were perhaps more than 300 students screaming and yelling and in various stages of loosing their minds. The police were still arriving and those who had arrived were doing their best to give Dave and me a place and a chance to work on this young lady who had just suffered what would turn out to be a fatal stab wound to her chest.

As we came to an abrupt stop about fifteen feet from the victim, I said to Dave, "just stay close to me, and for now just do what I tell you!"

As he nodded his head in agreement, I leaped out of the ambulance, opened the side doors, gave Dave the drug box, and I said, "When we get to her side, do you think you can set-up a lactated ringers IV for me?"

In about the most nervous voice I perhaps have ever heard he said, "Yeah, I think so."

I then grabbed the airway box and we hustled over to the side of our first of more than 2,000 patients that we would see over the next couple of years. I quickly assessed her condition and found her to be quite dead. Without hesitation, I got one of the police officers on the scene to do chest compressions for us. I then opened the airway box, removed the required equipment and intubated our patient. While I was doing that, Dave did set up the correct IV solution along with the correct tubing with it.

As he finished that, I had just finished intubating the patient and was securing the endotracheal tube to her face. I then placed the Ambu-bag to the end of the tube so we could breathe for her. As the screaming and chaos was escalating, I told Dave to trade places with me so he could do the rescue breathing and I could quickly get an IV started. Now wasn't the time to teach him or to let him "try". There is always a place and time to let the puppies play, but that wasn't it.

Just as I started a large bore IV, one of our basic ambulances arrived to give us some much-needed assistance on this call. I remember my two colleagues having to blow their sirens just to get the throngs of people out of their way to get to our side. As a relief, I saw my former partner Dave Hawkins, jump out of one side of the ambulance, and my good friend Bill Boyd on the other side.

As I looked back at the patient, I noticed my new partner, Dave kneeling at the head of our patient with Ambu-bag in hand, just looking at her with a wide-eyed stare, and not moving a single muscle. I couldn't believe it. He looked absolutely terrified and was just frozen.

Instinctively, I just yelled to him and said, "You can at least bag, can't ya?" Suddenly his eyes snapped up to me, and he vigorously shook his head yes. He looked back to our patient and started squeezing the bag for all he was worth.

"Easy does it!" I said. "Just squeeze it once every four or five seconds! That will do just fine!"

At that time, Hawkins is in my ear shouting at me, (so I can hear him) and asking me what I needed him and Bill to do. I asked Dave to take over ventilating the patient as Bill got the cot out of my ambulance. We needed to get this patient out of this out-of-control chaos and to the hospital, which was only about a dozen blocks away. Ingeson hurried to his feet to help Bill get the cot when he inadvertently hooked the IV tubing with one of his feet and proceeds to unknowingly rip the IV catheter out of the patient's arm. Life-sustaining fluid was spilling out onto the parking lot, the patient's arm was hemorrhaging, and everything was now contaminated.

After a few "!@#$%^" and a couple of "#$&*!," I restarted the IV. We then rolled and secured her onto a backboard and then lifted her onto our cot. The four of us swiftly loaded her into the ambulance and whisked her off to the hospital. I gave the job of ventilating the patient back to my new partner and my old partner drove us to the local emergency room just as fast as was possible.

As soon as we were underway to the hospital I radioed the emergency room and told them that we were en route with a teenaged black female with a single stab wound to her mid chest, just to the right of her sternum (breast bone). I told them that she was pulseless but we had her intubated and a large bore IV in place and that we were doing CPR; we would be hitting the doors at their facility in less than two minutes.

The ambulance came to a screeching halt at the hospitals'

emergency department and we quickly unloaded our patient and rushed her through the glass double doors. As we are turning the cot to the left and into the emergency room, one of the cardiac surgeons was running down the hallway right at us in a dead sprint. I will never forget the stern look on his face, his blue scrubs pulling hard across his body with every stride, his surgical mask hanging from his neck, and holding a scalpel high over his head.

In just a few seconds, the patient, paramedics, EMT's, emergency room staff, and the cardiac surgeon all met at a bed that was waiting for us. In just a matter of three or four seconds we had pulled from our cot the lifeless body of a teenager. The emergency staff took over the CPR, ventilating, and looked for yet another IV access point as the surgeon stood at her side.

As he looked down at her with unblinking and steely eyes, he immediately put his scalpel to her mid-chest and in less than a single second her chest was open from her sternum to a mid-point between her waist and armpit. In an instant, blood was gushing from the massive incision. It reminded me of someone just quickly pouring water out of a bucket and onto the floor. It was something I'll never forget.

The assailant's knife had severed a pulmonary artery. When the young lady hit the pavement, she was dying. When her heart finished pumping nearly every drop of blood from her cardiovascular system and into her chest cavity, she was finished. It wouldn't have mattered in the least whether the people who came to her aid that fateful day in the parking lot of a local high school were medical first responders or general surgeons, the result would be the same. She would have ended up just as dead. But that is beside the point.

Dave Ingeson went on to work for Medic 1 for five and a half years, and left to work for another ambulance company for another four years before getting into the nursing profession. He and I worked together as regular partners for roughly two years. I taught him what I could and he learned quickly. Although early on he made it a habit of running to the restroom when we were being dispatched to a serious call, he soon became a highly competent and effective paramedic. When he left Medic 1 in June 1988, on that day, he was as great of a paramedic as he was an inept one on his first day at Medic 1.

Today, the fresh out of school paramedics could (and should) enjoy the same internship that Dave Ingeson enjoyed. If current management was truly concerned about the level of competent patient care that we deliver today, management would say, "Hey, we know that you are new to this side of the EMS profession. We know that we don't have any right to expect that you should know it all, all at once. We know that taking what you've learned in the classroom and transferring it to real life situations in the street and on the fly is under the best of circumstances, very difficult.

"We know that we should give you the time that you and your patients whose life you may be altering and or saving the opportunity to learn under the tutelage and watchful eye of someone whose been there and done that. We know that at times you will have to deal with patients who have multi-system failures and traumas. We know that at times you will have to be jumping around the back end of your ambulance like a jack rabbit just to give your patient a fighting chance at survival. And above it all, we know that you will at sometime, make a mistake.

"It may be a benign mistake or it may be catastrophic. And we know that the mistake you are all but assured of making will most likely be somewhere in the middle. But we know, it will happen. We know this because we know that it happens to everybody. Sooner or later, it happens to everybody. We plainly know better, but that's not the way it's going to be, so deal with it."

The following are a few true accounts of what happens when puppies in the workplace are thrown to the dogs far too soon. The following are true accounts of what happens when management knows better but doesn't care enough about good, reputable, and competent patient care to do what they fully know is the right thing. It's about what happens when the people who are "calling the shots" are just not that concerned in the pre-hospital care that is delivered on a daily basis.

***

A call came in for a man in his late 30s with a medical history of insulin dependent diabetes complaining about a bad headache. The crew that was sent to his aid consisted of a really good basic EMT and a paramedic who has had a license for far less than six months. When they arrived, they found a man sitting on his bed who was alert and oriented. He did indeed have diabetes and he said that his head was just pounding. The two responders took a small sample of his blood and were able to measure his blood-glucose level.

Depending on who you listen to, most experts in the endocrinology field of medicine will tell you that the normal range for your blood-glucose level is between 70-110 mg./dl. of blood. His level was at 68. With any gluco-meter, there is a +/- error factor of anywhere between 2-5% percent. So in all actuality, his blood-glucose level should have been realized as being on the low side of normal. It wasn't. (Mistake #1).

On top of that, with the patient being alert and not the slightest bit lethargic or disoriented, it should have been recognized at that point the likelihood of it "not" being a diabetic problem.

It wasn't. (Mistake #2)

As a consequence the paramedic zeroed in on a "low blood sugar" problem rather than perhaps looking for another reason for his bad headache. (Mistake #3)

As a result of mistake #1, the paramedic decided to start an IV on the patient and gave him a 25-gram vial of dextrose, which shot his blood sugar to over 260mg./dl. of blood. (Mistake #4)

One of the "side effects" of giving dextrose is that it increases intra-cranial pressure. The increased pressure is a non-issue if there is no problem with the blood circulation within the brain.

Well as it turns out, the reason he had a headache in the first place was that he had been suffering from a brain hemorrhage. When the intra-cranial pressure increased so did the bleeding. This sent the patient into a seizure and the new paramedic running for the airway box.

Meanwhile the basic EMT was left there to maintain an airway as best as he could by using the jaw thrust method. When the paramedic returned to the scene of the screw-up, the EMT opened the airway box and inserted a nasopharyngeal airway to the patient to maintain a clear passage for his breathing.

In the meantime, the paramedic opened the drug box, and gets the Valium. By this time the patient had stopped seizing, but the paramedic gave the patient a 10mg. bolus of Valium anyway. (Mistake #5)

In short order, the patient's rate of respirations had decreased to eight to ten per minute. Now the patient needed respiratory support. Due to the depressive effects Valium has on the respiratory system, the Ambu-bag was used to support the patient's rate of respirations by forcing air into his lungs at a faster rate than he was currently breathing. Now the new paramedic turned his attention to the compromised airway of his patient and decided to intubate.

Over the objection and to the dismay of the EMT, the paramedic removed the nasopharyngeal airway that had just been inserted a few short minutes before and attempted endotracheal intubation. After the tube was inserted, the EMT listened for lung sounds and found them to be absent.

Unfortunately, there was plenty of air being pumped into the patient's stomach. When the EMT advised the paramedic of his findings, the paramedic said it "couldn't be", he was sure he saw the tube go between the vocal cords and into the trachea. Apparently it didn't. (Mistake #6).

Less than a minute later, stomach contents were shooting up through the tube that was just inserted. Now, the faulty placement of the endotracheal tube has caused what used to be a patent airway, now to become a highly compromised and dangerous airway in which the patient will invariably aspirate stomach contents into the lungs.

If the patient survives, it will invariably mean pneumonia and infection. Now the patient was just simply rushed to the hospital in a much worse condition than he was in prior to the arrival of the two pre-hospital healthcare providers. The eventual diagnosis this patient had was an intra-cranial hemorrhage.

The reason all of this happened isn't because the new paramedic wasn't educated properly or didn't care enough or whatever. The only thing that he was guilty of was a lack of working, field experience and that wasn't his fault. Without a doubt, the biggest error was his assignment to be working with a basic EMT. (Mistake #7)...Or was that mistake #1?

***

Another call came into our central station on an early Saturday afternoon, late spring day. This call for an ambulance was for a 2-year-old girl who had wandered out into the middle of a busy neighborhood street. Apparently she had followed her mother who had crossed the street to talk with a neighbor. The toddler ran out into the path of a car from between two parked cars and was struck.

When the "new" paramedic and the basic EMT arrived at the scene, they had with them a paramedic student doing some "ride time". The student is there with the ambulance crew to observe techniques, protocols and to observe the general operations of an advanced life support ambulance in the pre-hospital setting.

When the three of them arrived, they found a highly-chaotic scene with a crowd of forty to fifty people, including the mother of the child who had just been badly injured. Mom was in a verbal melee with her mother because grandma was assessing blame for the accident on the mother of the child.

There was just one police officer there when EMS arrived and the officer was doing her best in attempting to control the ever-increasing size of the crowd. Prior to the arrival of the ambulance someone had removed the unconscious child from the street and laid her in a nearby yard.

The child was found to be vacillating between a painful, crying lethargy and a non-breathing unconsciousness. Her legs were found to be splayed open. The "new" paramedic (after she did a quick head-to-toe assessment) thought correctly that the little girl might have suffered a pelvic fracture. Due to the severity of the call a second ambulance was dispatched to assist the primary ambulance if needed. That crew also had a paramedic student with them.

The basic EMT of the primary ambulance immediately knelt at the head of the patient and placed his hands on both sides of the child's head so as to stabilize her neck in the event of a possible cervical spine injury. At this time the second ambulance arrived along with the crew chief who came in yet a separate vehicle. The basic EMT at the head of the patient told the rider to retrieve a specialized backboard and cervical collar. The rider couldn't find the needed items. The EMT then sent one of the crew members from the second ambulance to bring the needed equipment. No problem.

After that, the same crew member from the second ambulance was asked by the attending EMT to interface with the toddler's mother so as to keep her out of the way. It cannot be understated just how important that is.

The child was then properly back boarded and then placed inside the ambulance. At that time the crew chief asked the EMT (not the paramedic) what he, the EMT, needed next. (The crew chief also knew instantly who the effective crew member on the first ambulance was.) The EMT stated to the crew chief that he needed lung sounds checked and then rapid transport to the local emergency room.

One of the paramedic students tried to check lung sounds but "couldn't hear much at all". (That's no surprise because students have very little idea on what normal lung sounds would sound like, let alone lung sounds of a compromised respiratory system due to traumatic injury.) At that point one of the other EMT's jumped into the driver's seat and sped the ambulance to the hospital. Now we have the lead EMT, the "new" paramedic and not one but two students in the back of the ambulance with a very seriously injured 2-year-old little girl.

The lead EMT alternated high-flow oxygen with a non-rebreather mask and then would have to assist her ventilations with the bag-valve-mask device (BVM) when her own breathing became less than adequate. That would be critical if this little girl would survive her ordeal. All the while the "new" paramedic is preoccupied with the little girl's legs. She tried to get a response from the patient by tapping the bottom of her feet. No vital signs were obtained. The heart monitor was not placed on the patient. Lastly, no IV access was attempted. All of this was extremely important, yet none of it was done.

Every pre-hospital healthcare provider—be that MFR, EMT, Specialist or Paramedic—has to know what is and what is not important on each call. You learn that through experience gleaned from working with experienced healthcare providers. That little girl and her family can thank God that an experienced basic EMT was first on the scene. It's just a shame that the company didn't have a paramedic "calling the shots" who knew what was important, instead of a basic EMT who couldn't and shouldn't be responsible for emergency health care that can be a matter of life and death when a paramedic is present.

There are scores of examples both large and small just like this. Minor snafus to major screw-ups have happened. All of these examples are not stated to impugn the honest efforts of new paramedics and their best efforts to help people who may be badly injured or desperately ill. Quite the opposite. I know from first hand experience the pressures that are felt. To know in your heart of hearts, that you cannot reasonably handle this type of call or that type of emergency call is something you don't want to experience. To know that you'll need help and that help will in all likelihood not be available has to be just a little disconcerting.

With all of this being said, Medic 1 Ambulance is still a great place to work if you want to test yourself, and become a paramedic in more than name only. Due to the sheer number of calls that you will respond to on a daily, monthly, and yearly rate, it's a great place for professional development. The number of emergency calls generated here at Medic 1 dwarfs those by other nearby professional companies, not to mention the handful of volunteer services still in operation.

The only good thing to come from this type of baptism by fire is that if you have the propensity, fortitude and inner strength to succeed and ultimately be successful, then you may just become a good and effective paramedic. If you have leadership qualities in addition to the aforementioned attributes, you may even become a great paramedic. Within a year, you as well as those around you will know.

Chapter 7
STICKS AND STONES

When I got into the EMS business, I had no real idea of the kind of mind set that would allow people to think so little of their neighbors, their families, or even themselves. But over many years, I have witnessed bigotry, hatred, ignorance, contempt for authority, and apathy that plagues far too many people in the cities and towns of these United States. There is the one thing that I absolutely cannot, and have not come to grips with. Those are the times when we, as emergency medical care providers, are summoned to render emergency medical support and find ourselves the victims of attack.

Where I grew up was not unlike a Norman Rockwell picture. Although I lived in an agriculturally-based community, the small quaint little town that it surrounded was for the most part quiet. Between the two entities a little more than 5,500 people call this place home. The area still has at last count eight different churches and had until recently at least four public places that served open intoxicants.

On top of that, the local city police department was at one time just a couple of guys who might remind you of Andy and Barney from the 1960s series, *The Andy Griffin Show*. The county sheriff's department covered the township. Today, the city and the township each have their own police departments with several full and part-time officers.

The violence that is so prevalent in the larger towns and big cities for the most part was a fairly alien notion to most of the people who I grew up with. I'm not talking about the violent collisions and associated carnage that is associated with high velocity planes, trains, and various kinds of automobiles. And I'm surely not talking about the fights that occur now and again on the grammar school playground anymore than when old "Hank" gets drunk and knocks around his wife. I'm talking about the cycles of violence and abuses that people in some communities perpetrate on each other that result in great bodily injury or death.

While I was growing up in a two-parent household, about the only real violence I saw was the violence on the six o'clock news. As far as I was concerned, that kind of mayhem was an abstract thought. I never saw or heard of anyone who was shot, stabbed, or bludgeoned to death.

As someone who (thankfully) never had to live that lifestyle, the thought of that kind of violence was something that happened to other people in other places. It didn't happen here, and it sure didn't happen to me. As far as I was concerned, there was no doubt in my mind that because I grew up in a two-parent family, I have been blessed with both love and security.

Thankfully, none of my three children know what it is like to have to live each day with the threat of some kind of violence. Anything is possible, but I'm comparing my community with the neighborhoods where the sounds of crying children, screaming women, gunshots, and the sirens of emergency vehicles are an everyday event.

On occasion when EMS providers enter some homes in some of these communities (to render simple first-aid or life saving advanced life support intervention), we find ourselves on the wrong end of a gun, a knife, a fist, or boot. Too many times we find that we ourselves are seeking medical attention for wounds suffered because some out of control, half-witted moron sees us as the enemy, or just feels that he (or she) has to strike out at somebody for whatever reason. Too often EMS personnel are an easy, as well as a defenseless target.

Even though it has happened, it is exceedingly rare that EMS providers ever wear body armor or carry any kind of weapon. Despite the fact that we go into some of the most chaotic and dangerous places and situations, we see ourselves as those who are there simply to give aid, comfort, and help to those in need of various levels of medical care. We are not there to detain, arrest, or jail anyone and therefore we don't pose any kind adverse relationship to anybody.

Normally, EMS providers don't pass judgment, or even criticize those people in need of medical care or treatment. We don't do it, even though by most standards some of these people richly deserve to be screamed at. Right or wrong, I do pass judgment or criticize people who abuse the service I provide when they don't *need* my services, or simply use me as a simple and expedient transportation tool. My frustrations are more global in that the public service provided has become adulterated for an unintended use…convenience. This is absolutely not what the public should pay for.

So it really irritates me to the point of near madness when I'm assaulted in any physical fashion. As a result, I go to a mental and emotional place or state of mind that is rooted in an expectation of at least a minimal amount of respect (if not appreciation for the uniform I wear and the profession I represent).

Accordingly, in the event of a physical confrontation, I will react harshly in a verbal manner and sometimes in a physical method in order to avoid, or preempt the real possibility of serious personal injury to me or my partner. If a weapon is involved, I will do anything that gets us out of immediate danger—no matter what that may entail. For me, it's a survival mentality that I make no apologies for.

Consequently, I don't have a single problem with beating the stuffing out of someone who has, for no apparent reason, attacked me or any of my partners. Of the more than 35,000 ambulance calls over the last three decades, violence, and the very real threat of violence perpetrated on EMS providers, is a working condition that is all too real.

***

The very first time I ran into a violent situation was when I had just started to work for Medic 1 Ambulance. I had only been working for perhaps a month when we received a call to back up another one of our ambulances. They were involved with an extremely violent male in his mid-to-late 20s. As I remember, the individual had just "flipped-out" when his mother had unexpectedly passed away.

We later learned that this guy never had a dad, one of his brothers was in prison, his only sister had been raped weeks earlier, and who knows what else he had been dealing with. Apparently, when his mom passed on, that was just the straw that broke the camel's back.

When my partner Donny Cronk and I arrived in the predominately African-American neighborhood, it was to the scene of something that—up until that moment in time—I had never before witnessed. It was total unbridled mayhem. There were perhaps more than 300 people yelling and screaming for a variety of reasons. About half of them wanted us gone immediately! The other half wanted us to hurry along faster than we were able.

There were several squad cars and maybe a dozen police officers from two to three different departments who were not being warmly greeted. In addition, Donny and I were getting pushed around by some of those in the throng of people present, and bottles, bricks, and stones were heading our way. In the middle of it all are two of my colleagues, Ray Horton and Mike Schultz, who were fighting along with at least three or four police officers, all trying to subdue one very strong and disturbed individual. The man was filled with hatred for the law, authority, and the rage of a life unraveling.

As we got there, Mike saw Donny and me coming and yelled over the near deafening noise of the crowd to get our ambulance cot. We immediately turned around and hustled the forty yards back to where our ambulance was parked. We retrieved our cot, and now had to run the same gauntlet a second time, this time with an ambulance cot in tow.

We again arrived at the patient's side as the police officers involved with the melee (along with Mike and Ray) had just gotten the "flipped out" individual hand-cuffed and lying prone on the ground. All five of them—including the patient—looked like they just went through a meat grinder. The clothes on each of them were ripped and dirty. There were scrapes, abrasions, and minor cuts all around. And since it was a very hot summer day, everybody was pouring sweat out by the buckets.

The four of us who were there as EMS providers, picked the kicking and screaming patient up from the ground and laid him in a prone position on our ambulance cot. We tied him to it. I remember this guy attempted to get himself loose while screaming death threats to all of us. He had plenty of fight left in him.

The four of us each had a corner of the cot so he wouldn't tip the cot over while we were rolling it over in the broken glass and rock-strewn yard toward the ambulance. The police officers were doing their best to give us room by pushing, threatening, or cajoling the crowd to cooperate and to stay out of the way. I felt at the time it would have taken the smallest of insults, an unnecessary push or verbal abuse to send about half of the crowd into a violent frenzy.

As we are traversing our way through the throngs of mostly hostile people, we were still being shoved, spit on, sworn at, and so forth.

After we loaded our patient into the back of our ambulance, I watched Mike and Ray start to walk toward their ambulance. With people still yelling and screaming at them, a man came up from behind, reached out and grabbed Mike by his shoulder just as he is reaching for the door handle on the ambulance. He viciously spun him around, and Mike followed through with a well-planted fist to this guy's face. Mike hit him so hard that for an instant the man was in a horizontal position, about four-feet high off the ground. The man hit the ground in a heap.

At the same time, one of the Benton Harbor city police officer's came over to this guy lying on the ground. While Mike was getting into his ambulance, the city cop (who was African American) looked down at this guy, kicked him and said, "You won't fuck with that white boy next time, will ya'?"

I thought to myself, "Holy Christ, I'm in 1880, Dodge City!"

***

A couple of years later, I was working with a very fine paramedic named Bob Ristau. He and I received a call about 11 p.m. for a woman who had passed out. As we pulled up to the scene, we found a house that was completely dark. Bob grabbed his flashlight and I grabbed our airway box, blood pressure cuff, and stethoscope. We exited the ambulance and walked briskly from the street curb up to the house. We knocked on the door and in a few seconds it quickly opened to a man who said that his girlfriend had "fell out."

We entered the house and although it was late at night, there were no lights on in the house. Other than Bob's flashlight, the only other light was what was coming through a living room window from a distant streetlight. Bob illuminated the living room where this woman was lying supine on the floor. After looking at her for just a moment, I could tell that she was breathing adequately, and after a few more seconds I found her blood pressure and heart rate were just fine. I also found her to be faking her unconscious condition.

I have never understood why some people will fake this type of thing and cause other people to get the emergency services involved. When supposed adults choose to act in such a childish or juvenile manner it just smacks of intellectual ignorance and immaturity. Unfortunately, this type of "acting out" is all too common and it has always really irritated me.

After assessing her and finding her to be quite awake, I should have told Bob in a coded way that this particular woman was faking. We now do this often by saying things like "we have feigned syncope here" or " we have a thespian here" or "we have prompted-eye flutter here," or something in that fashion.

I said, "Hey, I mean no disrespect but this woman here is faking. She can hear everything we are saying and if she wanted to, she could get right up off the floor."

Well those few words of honest assessment were apparently not the thing to say. Immediately the other two men and three women in the house became incensed with my statement. They vehemently questioned my conclusion along with my integrity. One man was so upset that he grabbed a butcher knife and started threatening us.

He didn't thrust the knife at either of us, but he did brandish it and said, "I'm going to cut your white asses!"

I saw the blade but Bob didn't. I just blurted out, "Bob, he's got a knife! He's got a knife!"

Bob yelled, "Where? Where?" as he moved his flashlight all around the room trying to find which person had the weapon.

It only took my partner a few moments to quickly find the man who was threatening us with his knife. Bob and I had the front door at our back.

"Easy man," I said calmly, just trying to get towards the door. "We're going to go out and get our cot from the ambulance."

At that instant, we hustled out of the house and not looking behind us, we flat out ran to the ambulance. As we got inside our vehicle, I reached for the radio to call our dispatcher, and while trying to catch our breath, I told him what had happened and that we needed the police immediately. As I was talking to our dispatcher, Bob wheeled the ambulance around and focused all of our spotlights, headlights, and load lights onto the house that we just escaped from. Within a minute or two, we had squad cars speeding our way from every direction.

Once they arrived, we told the officers that a man in the house had threatened us with a knife. They went into the house first and within a few seconds we could see the flicker of several flashlights and could hear the sounds of scuffling. Within a minute the officers had somebody handcuffed, and were haphazardly dragging him from the house.

Although I didn't get a good look at the man's face (as I was too busy staring at the knife he was holding), I knew immediately from his clothing that they had the wrong man in custody.

"That's not him! He's not the one who had the knife! He's still inside the house!"

One officer stayed outside with the man they had just dragged out while the other three or four officers along with Bob and me, went back inside and quickly found our perpetrator hiding under a bed. Within a second or two they had turned the bed over and had snatched up the guy lying on the floor.

While being pulled from under the bed by his feet, he started shaking and pretending to have a seizure. The cops eased him back onto the floor where he continued his "shaking."

As I witness this fictitious malady I became immediately incensed and shouted out, "He's a faking son-of-a-bitch! There's not a goddamn thing wrong with him that a good ass-kicking wouldn't fix!"

Without missing a beat, the woman—who up until this minute was lying on the floor pretending to be unconscious—leaped to her feet and grabbed a bottle of prescription medicine that happened to be setting on a table. She declared, "I'm a nurse! I'm a nurse and I know what to do!"

She then proceeds to pop the top off of the prescription bottle, straddled the man on the floor, and sat on his chest. Without hesitation, she pours capsules of what turned out to be the drug Dilantin (used to suppress seizures) out of the bottle and into the man's mouth. After witnessing this, one of the police officer's looks at me with a quizzical expression on his face, and as I look back at him I just shrugged my shoulders and gave him one of those: "I couldn't care less what happens to this guy" looks.

"Jim, should she be doing that?" one cop asked me.

"No, but don't worry. We'll pick up the pieces when she's done overdosing him. Besides, can't you tell...she's a 'nurse'?"

The self-proclaimed nurse looked up at me and shouted, "Fuck you! I am a nurse!"

"Yeah right, and I'm Santa Claus," I shot back. "Besides, what do you know? You were unconscious just thirty seconds ago. What I know for sure is that you certainly aren't a lady. Now get your ass off of him!"

As soon as I said that, the police officer grabbed her arm and sternly pulled her away from our latest faker. Without hesitation, Bob reached down and grabbed him by the collar and said, "All right you son-of-a-bitch, get on your feet!"

Of course he wouldn't move his legs let alone his feet. I said to him, "Listen you asshole, we know you can hear us and we know you're trying to bullshit us, and we know your trying to keep your dumb ass out of jail! What you don't know is that's its not working! Now knock it off and start walking!"

The guy got up and began stumbling around like he was attempting to gets his wits about him. Bob and I didn't buy it one minute. So each of us grabbed him under his arms and dragged him out of the house, across the yard, and we launched him from the street and onto the floor of the ambulance.

Once in the ambulance I jumped into the patient compartment. I really got into his face and called him about every name in the book. I also told him just how lucky he was that we only had to drive a minute or two to the hospital, because had it been longer, he would have been in for the beating of a lifetime. Of course he just laid there and ridiculously pretended that he was unconscious, or didn't hear me, or some such thing.

We drove him the six or eight blocks to the hospital, stopped the ambulance, opened the back doors, and dragged the man out of the ambulance and into the emergency room. After releasing him to the hospital, one of the officers took our report. He told us that since the guy didn't actually lunge at us in a bona fide attempt to stab or cut either of us, it wouldn't be worth our trouble to pursue prosecution. At the time I thought that it was a sad state of affairs that somebody could clearly threaten your life and that since there wasn't an actual attempt at murdering either Bob or myself, that it would be deemed not worthwhile as far as law enforcement, and the judicial systems were concerned.

The officer did go into the emergency room and to the bed where our perpetrator was lying. He told him he was extremely fortunate that Bob and I decided not to press charges for assault with intent to murder, because he would be facing ten to fifteen years behind bars. While this fictitious story is being told by this highly trained and experienced police officer to this mental half-pint, Bob and I are standing outside and around the corner of the room he's lying in, just quietly laughing our asses off. I guess after having the hell scared out of you by someone wanting to run you through with a butcher's knife just a short twenty minutes before, the good laugh we were both having was cathartic.

After a good five-minute ass chewing was concluded by the police officer, he came out of the emergency room from where this patient was laying. As he approached us, he saw that we were just busting a gut.

"You liked that didn't you?" he asks with a sheepish grin on his face.

"Oh man! That was great!" Bob said.

"Well if nothing else, he won't be bothering you guys again."

After thinking about that last statement by the police officer; it was all that Bob and I really wanted in the first place.

***

Once in awhile, you just know that a call is going to be nothing but trouble. Such was the case where my then partner Carl Brasier and I responded to a call that came in for a patient who had been involved in a bar fight, but was now at his home and apparently in need of an ambulance. We responded to the man's house in a timely manner and found that a single squad car from the local fire department was already there. As we entered the house, we found the local fire chief talking with a man in his mid 20s, who appeared heavily intoxicated. He was leaning with most of his weight against a wall with one of his hands straight up over his head.

The guy had been drinking at the local American Legion Hall. It was unclear whether he had been intoxicated upon his arrival at that establishment or whether he became inebriated during his stay. At some point the man reportedly became very belligerent, obnoxious and confrontational with the bartender and other patrons. According to witnesses, personal hostilities escalated up until the man was picked up off of his feet and was physically thrown out of the legion hall landing shoulder first on the cement sidewalk.

I don't recall now how our patient got to his home about three miles from the American Legion Hall, but whatever the case, he came home instead of going to the emergency room. Who knows why? To complicate the issue, the fire chief was his father. So now we have a man who has a few scrapes, an injured shoulder and who appears to be intoxicated to the point that it wouldn't have surprised me if he passed out.

Part of me would have preferred that he was unconscious because with his loud and obnoxious swearing, spewing of profanities and epithets, it is obvious that he is as just as mad as hell at the whole world. In short, other than urinating on himself, he was being just as nasty and disgusting as he possibly could.

His father (who was supposed to be acting as a medical first responder) was acting more like a really pissed off father than a professional firefighter. He was stomping around yelling about those "goddamn guys at the legion," and at the same time being as mad as hell at his son.

The two of them were yelling and raising hell with each other. In retrospect, after seeing all of this, Carl or I should have called for at least one police officer to come to the scene of our father-son reunion. Unfortunately, I would regret that lack of foresight. Carl and I had walked right in the middle of a bad situation.

After we got the pertinent history of what and how the incident happened, I attempted to examine and manipulate the injured man's shoulder. It was important to assess blood supply to his hand and arm as well as a range of motion to his injured shoulder. It should have been fairly simple but when I touched his shoulder to examine it, he instantly became extremely verbally abusive.

"Don't touch me you mother fucker, or I'll beat your mother fucking ass!" He said no less than a dozen times over the next fifteen minutes. The first time he said that I told him in no uncertain terms that the only reason I was touching him at all was that it was my job. I was there to help him and that involved an examination, which was extremely hard to do without touching him. I told him to calm down and quiet down. He did neither.

I turned to the fire chief and said, "You know, I really don't need this at all. Since his legs work just fine, why don't you just walk him out to your squad car and take him to the hospital yourself?"

"No by God! That's what you're here for and you're going to take him," he blurted back.

Had I not been in my 20s, I would have told his loud-mouthed father that if he thought I was going to take his booze-soaked and near-violent son to the hospital, he had another thing coming. But I was pretty much a young kid myself and I didn't have anywhere near the experience that I have now.

On our way out to the ambulance to retrieve our cot, both Carl and I thought that his father should be the one taking him to the local emergency room. Carl even mentioned that the patient in his present condition and demeanor was going to be nothing but trouble. But neither of us at the time thought that we could change his father's mind. So a few seconds later we were back in the house with the cot and proceeded to unfold the blanket and sheet.

We then invited him to sit down and then lie down so we could get him properly covered and shield him from the inclement weather. Surprisingly, he got onto the cot without much acrimony or fanfare. We told him to lie still as not to aggravate any injury that he may have sustained from being launched out of the local American Legion Hall. We wheeled him out to the ambulance, lifted him and the cot into the back of the ambulance, and made him as comfortable as possible.

After I climbed into the back of the ambulance, Carl shut the back doors, jumped in behind the steering wheel, and proceeded to drive to the local hospital. We hadn't traveled a mile when the patient started to squirm and was soon kicking the blanket and sheet off of him and onto the floor of the ambulance. In less than three minutes, he had unbuckled the cot straps and was sitting on the ambulance stretcher with his feet on the floor.

All the while, I attempted (in vain) to keep him calm and still and all the while talking in a very low key, gentle, and soft manner. The more I talked to him in that soft, calm, and reassuring tone, the more angry and obnoxious he became. He even said that unless I turned off the lights in the patient compartment of the ambulance, he was going to "kick my mother fucking ass."

I certainly didn't turn the lights off, but I did turn them down to the lowest setting possible. Still that didn't make him happy. Finally, I said to him, "If you don't want to hurt yourself further, you're going to have to get your feet back onto the cot and lay still!"

"Fuck you!" was his response.

Then completely out of the blue, in a roundhouse manner, he hit me with his fist, squarely on the middle of my chest with his full weight. The impact of his punch caused me to slide on the bench seat on which I was sitting. The swift and sudden impact of his punch really startled me. Almost as a reflex action and in an instant I thought that if I don't do something immediately, I might get the hell kicked out of me.

So I punched him in a jabbing type of punch and hit him in the middle of his forehead. He fell back face up onto the cot just as I was getting to my feet. He has crossed a line that caused me to have to defend myself. By striking out at him, I know he has caused me a whole lot of trouble. However, I wanted him to know that when he crossed the line from verbal threats to a physical assault, that he would have no doubt that I would have none of it.

And as such I yelled at him, "Alright you asshole, you wanna dance? Let's dance!"

After a few more choice words to him, instantly his demeanor changed.

"Oh man, I'm sorry, I'm sorry. I don't know why I just did that. I'm sorry," he said pleading forgiveness.

I then committed the cardinal sin. I took my eyes off and turned my head away from someone who had just punched me as hard as he could in the chest. All of a sudden, I was hit with another roundhouse punch on the left side of my neck. My eyeglasses flew off of my face, the back of my head hit the sidewall of the ambulance, and I was momentarily dazed, disoriented, and heading to the floor.

As I was going down, I could see my attacker getting to his feet. Instantly, I jabbed at him and caught him with a lucky punch. Now he was going down and I was scrambling to my feet. Again, he was on his back and lying on the cot. This time, there was no apology forthcoming. But that was okay by me because I wasn't interested in listening to any of his crap anyway. I then drew back and I delivered a measured punch and knocked him unconscious and slightly bloodied his lip.

At the time, it wasn't necessarily my intention to render him unconscious, but I wanted to let him know that I wasn't about to just merely stand here and trade punches with him any longer. My sole intention was to end this fight before I got hurt. (Days later, I was telling my story of the incident to another emergency room doctor by the name of James O. Galles. He stated that I was probably fortunate that I was struck on the side of the neck as opposed to my throat. The doctor said that with that much force, the idiot who was my patient, could have fractured my larynx and quite possibly could have killed me.)

By the time we arrived at the hospital about ten minutes later, my patient was again awake and as mad as hell. That was all right with me because I was just a little more than irritated myself. When Carl and I pulled the cot out of the ambulance with him on it, I remember distinctly telling him, "If you hit me again, I'm going to kill you right here and right now!"

Maybe he thought that I might just be half serious or perhaps he had thought that he was in enough trouble already. For whatever reason, he was well behaved as we moved him out of the hospital's ambulance garage, into the emergency room and onto one of their beds. He wasn't my problem anymore.

I was told later that in just a few short minutes, he was up and running around the emergency room. It took several hospital security guards, two police officers and high dose of Vistaril (a drug that at one time was given intramuscularly for the acutely disturbed or hysterical patient) to keep him under control.

After Carl and I wheeled our patient into the emergency room and took him from our cot to the hospital bed, I told the attending physician what had transpired over the previous twenty-five minutes. He looked at me with one of those expressions that said: I've seen and heard this before from EMS providers. But he just said, "Jim, I wouldn't have your job for any money."

The next day, I received a call at my home from one of my colleagues who worked with me at Medic 1, by the name of Mike Schultz. At the time of his call, Mike was working in the emergency room on a part-time basis. When I answered the phone he was almost whispering when he said to me,

"Hey Stiner, you know that guy you brought to the E.R. yesterday—that you got into the fight with?"

"Yeah, what about it?"

"Well he's back and the whole left side of his face is swollen and pushed out of shape. In fact, he can't even put a pair of sunglasses on. He's telling the doctor that someone hit him in the face with a flashlight. You didn't hit him with your light, did you?"

I was almost exasperated when I answered him. "Hell no! I didn't hit him with my flashlight! Maybe somebody else did, but I sure didn't!"

"He's saying that he thinks maybe the ambulance driver hit him in the face with a flashlight."

"No Mike, I hit him with my left hand, three times with measured punches. And besides, I was defending myself."

"I don't know Stine, his face really looks bad. You should see his x-rays. He's got several fractures."

At the time I thought that perhaps he had been hit with a flashlight, a pipe, or some such thing. I didn't think for a moment that I had struck him with my fist with sufficient force to cause multiple fractures of any kind. After the incident, I didn't have a single bruise or scratch on my hand at all. I had no pain whatsoever from striking him. I suppose it's nice to think you may have a punch that rivals one that is delivered by the likes of a Joe Louis or a Mike Tyson, but that's not really the case. So although he had fractures where I did strike him, it still wouldn't have surprised me in the least (on account of his attitude) that somebody got to him before I did.

Of course when something out of the ordinary happens such as this type of call, there is always an incident report that must be written about what out of the ordinary has occurred. I was very truthful and honest about what had happened and took responsibility for my actions. The paradox is that I probably let someone else off the hook by stating my actions. That was and still is okay with me because that's how I was raised. I believe strongly in honesty, integrity, and responsibility, even if it means that you may end up in some trouble later for a decision you've made.

After an investigation and reports, the guy filed an assault charge against me. On my behalf, Medic 1 filed similar charges with the county prosecutor's office against the plaintiff. The prosecutor refused to charge either of us with a crime, but a civil case was filed for pain and suffering. They asked for $50,000, but settled out of court for $30,000.

In turn, I also received a nasty letter from by boss that was deposited in my personnel file stating I used "poor judgment" while defending myself. I remember vehemently arguing with my boss about the content of the letter. As far as I know, it's still in the file. About the only thing I told him that he should know is that if the same set of circumstances happened in exactly the same way, I wouldn't hesitate to defend myself in the same manner.

It's always irritated me that pencil pushers, bureaucrats or people such as that who wouldn't dream of doing this type of work, rule in the abstract from their ivory towers. They always seem to think they know better than those people who are on the front lines and are doing the job on a daily basis. The trouble is that most Monday morning quarterbacks never played the game.

***

Another time that I got into a bit of a fracas was when my good friend Mike Schultz and I were working together. This is the same Mike that flattened the guy with a roundhouse punch to the face that I talked about earlier in this chapter. This time Mike came to my rescue. Mike and I had received a call about someone who had allegedly been assaulted. The information we had been told was that someone had been kicked and punched primarily in the ribs. According to our dispatcher, there wasn't any life threatening problems. We left the station and drove to this young man's residence in a normal rate of speed that was consistent with the other traffic on the streets so we didn't' need to use our emergency lights or sirens.

Our slow arrival had upset the man who appeared to be in his early 20s. We found him lying on his uninjured side. As I approached him, I asked where he hurt the most. No answer. I then said to him, "Hey, can you hear me?"

In a tone that was just as nasty as could be he says to me, "Yeah, I can hear ya' and it took you mother-fuckers long enough to get here!"

For a moment I was sort of confused by his comment. It had only taken us six minutes to get there. I then looked back at his father and he chimed in by saying to his son, "Hey don't say that. These men are here to help you." Again, no answer.

As I kneeled to assess him Mike asked the father if there were any other medical issues we should know about. I touched his rib cage and without hesitation, or a yell or a "that hurts," he threw his elbow back at me and hit me right in the nose. In an instant I was sitting on the floor with blood pouring out of my nose.

It took me a second or two to get my wits about me and I scrambled to my feet and yelled out, "Goddamn it! You stupid ass!" I then stomped out of the house and into the back of the ambulance to get myself cleaned up and to get something to plug my nose with. Mike came out immediately after me and asked me if I was okay. I assured him I was fine and told him to go get the patient ready for transport.

The thought of calling the police did cross my mind for a moment. However, a complaint of assault would have gone nowhere mostly because he would have argued that I surprised him by touching his injured ribs or that I hurt him further by placing my hands on him and that his actions were purely reflexive and not intentional. In the end, the whole incident would have been ruled an accidental punch in the nose, although we both knew that wasn't the case. In my mind, it was just another shot at EMS taken by someone who thought they needed to strike out at an easy target.

The father and son came out to the ambulance, and without a hint of an apology, the son climbed into the back of the ambulance with me and sits on the bench seat where I proceed to record his vital signs. Mike and the father sat in the front waiting for me to finish and give the okay to head to the hospital.

As we're moving down the street I did all I could to avoid talking to this man who just bloodied my nose and directed all of my questions to the father. At this time, I noticed that my patient was now lying down on the bench seat. I informed him that if his ribs were hurting that he has to sit up to breathe.

Instead of just pushing himself up by pushing off the bench seat, he reaches up to where he sees two small Velcro straps hanging down from the ceiling of the ambulance. The straps are used to secure IV bags in place so they don't swing wildly while the ambulance is moving and are little more than shoestrings. Before I could say a word or attempt to stop him, he had pulled them off of the ceiling.

In a fit of anger I said to him, "Hey pinhead, you elbowed me in the face, bloodied my nose, ruined my shirt and now you've broken the straps to my IV hanger! Is there anything else you could manage to do?"

"Yeah, there is!" he said as he lunged at me.

As thoughts ran through my mind, one was that there's not much wrong with his ribs if he's able and ready to fight again. I immediately fell back onto the attendant's chair and while he lunged, I kicked him in the chest. The force of the kick threw him toward the back of the ambulance. He lunged at me again and again and each time he got a size eleven boot to the chest.

During this brief little melee, this guy with the "rib pain" lunged at me a total of four times in a span of about fifteen seconds. Mike hit the brakes hard and slammed the transmission into park, which subsequently knocked this guy off of his feet and onto the bench seat. Mike came through the bulkhead of the ambulance (the portal between the cab and the patient compartment in an ambulance), and tackled the guy and pinned him to the bench seat. Mike suggested I drive and I didn't argue.

We hadn't gone a quarter mile down the street and Mike had warned the young man not to hit him as he eased off of holding him down to allow him to sit up. No sooner than Mike let him sit up, the patient attacked Mike and resumed his fighting. Before I could stop the ambulance, Mike had thrown him out through the back doors of the ambulance.

I remember looking at my rearview mirror and seeing the two back doors wide open. As I looked at my side view mirrors, I saw this guy that used to be our patient, tumbling down the street. To be honest, I had been slowing down because I had a stop sign about fifty yards in front of me and it was right at the hospital.

"You had better get out and get your son because we are done with him!" I said to his father.

"Boys, I'm sorry about all of this," he said embarrassed at his son's actions.

"Yeah, I'm sorry about it too. Good luck. You've got your hands full with him," I said.

Mike didn't bother with checking on this tumbling moron. Mike and this idiot's father passed each other as Mike jumped into the front passenger seat of the ambulance. As we pulled into the hospital's emergency entrance and parked our rig, Mike and I could still hear the son screaming and cussing at us—and at his father. He was making all kinds of threatening gestures and inviting us to fight with him and so on. From that point on, I figured that if he did actually get beat up, he richly deserved every punch, bite, scratch or kick he received.

Because of the nature of the job at Medic 1 Ambulance, the number of fights, wrestling matches and the like, that I had gotten involved in became so numerous that after awhile, it got to be no big deal. After I had gotten myself into all kinds of trouble by defending myself in the back of my ambulance by allegedly causing fractures to the guy I mentioned earlier, my partner Dave Ingeson and I decided to go out and buy a pair of handcuffs.

We thought although there was some ambiguity in the law about restraining patients (there were times when it was permitted to forcibly restrain your patient and there were times when it was pro-hibited), and because Medic 1 to this day still has no written policy on defense of one's self against a physical assault, if I or whoever I was working with felt threatened, then the patient will go in handcuffs or they wouldn't go at all. After getting myself knocked around in the back of the ambulance a few times, that was just the way it was going to be.

Frankly, at the time, I couldn't have cared less whether the boss or the powers that be liked it or not. The most important thing as far as I was concerned, (and I still strongly believe this) is my safety as well as the safety of my partner. All else is a distant second. As the old saying goes, "I'd rather be judged by twelve than carried by six."

When I had responded to crime scenes that involved violence, my handcuffs were always close by. People who were involved in drunken brawls where either one or both of the combatants were injured, the one who I took to the hospital, not always but often, got handcuffed. More than one time, I received enquiries from my patients as to why they were going to the local hospital wearing handcuffs since they were not under arrest. Sometimes, there would understandably be some resentment as well as resistance.

When some of the people became acutely argumentative and somewhat combative, I would simply say, "Do you see the way you are acting right now? Since you were involved in fighting (or whatever), you are going in handcuffs, because I don't feel like fighting with you. And believe me; the handcuffs you are wearing are for your protection. Because if for whatever reason you hit me, we're going to fight. And if we fight, you are going to come out on the short end of the stick. So just lay still until we get to the hospital and everything will be just fine."

About 99% of the time, that took care of any potential problems. If for whatever reason I had a female patient who had been involved in a violent encounter where she may have been the one that initiated the ensuing problem, I wouldn't handcuff her. At least a half dozen times, I should have. In each of those times, I would get hit, slapped or kicked by our patient. In each of those times I would simply say, "If you don't act like a lady, I'm not going to treat you like a lady!" That always took care of that particular problem.

Each of them, I think instinctively knew that they were going to receive the same treatment that their male counterparts would be getting if they would assault me again. The only difference between the two sexes is that for women, I would give them a stern and clear warning of what would happen if they were to strike me again. As for the men, they would be in for a fight. And if it were to take me, as well as my partner to restrain and bring our patient under control, then that's what it would take.

Now all of this is for the relatively few times that the police would not be at the scene of where we would be having a problem or for whatever reason, they had already left the scene or were busy with other aspects of our incident. Most of the time, if I felt I needed somebody handcuffed, they would already be handcuffed.

In the last few years, the violence perpetrated on me and most of the paramedics and EMT's that work at Medic 1 hasn't been to the degree that it once was. I don't know if it's because we live in a kinder and gentler community, or perhaps the police are much more visible and therefore the people who would otherwise commit a crime of violence on us have a second thought. I don't think anyone knows for sure. For all I know, it may be that it's because most of the "fun" people are either dead or in prison. In any case, I'm glad of it.

***

One of the more hair-raising ordeals I had been through happened several years ago. I was working with a guy by the name of Jim Mackey. Jim and I had been dispatched to a call involving a man with a gun, threatening suicide. As usual the county sheriff's department had been dispatched. For once, Jim and I had arrived on scene before the police. When we pulled up to the house, we noticed that there was a car in the driveway and the front door was ajar. We knocked on the partially opened door and not hearing anyone answer, yelled, "Hello, Medic 1!" Other than the ambulance engine running, we didn't hear a thing. We didn't want to go much further.

Jim and I hadn't been there but maybe a minute or two when County Deputy Sheriff Dave Chandler arrived. We briefly told him that we had just arrived and we knocked on the already open door and then yelled out, but heard nothing.

Dave said, "Well, let me go in first and see what is going on."

So he walks up to the door, knocks, calls out. Still no answer. We were all thinking that he was lying on the floor dead with a gunshot wound to the head or some such thing, that he was waiting for someone to walk through the door so he could "take somebody with him" kind of thing, or better, maybe nobody was home.

Dave was about as nervous as he could be when he entered the house. In fact, he pulled his service pistol about halfway out of his holster, and then put it back twice before he finally pulled it out totally as he went through the door. He instructed us to stay put until he found something. We had no problem with his orders. The whole thing just had a bad feel to it.

Within thirty seconds the deputy sheriff yelled, "Guys, get in here! Hurry, get in here!"

With a trauma box in my hand and my partner with an oxygen bottle and drug box in his hands, we hurried in and found a man in his early to mid-30s sitting upright on a couch. There was a coffee table in front of the couch with an array of scattered newspapers on the table and on the floor between the couch and the coffee table. The room itself looked like a relatively large family room.

It appeared he had shot himself in the chest during a suicide attempt, with a 9-mm Browning semi-automatic pistol. His wound was at about the fourth or fifth rib and about eight centimeters to the right side of his sternum. As I approached our patient it was obvious that he had a self-inflicted chest wound. The shirt had a small, round hole over the right breast and there was a considerable amount of blood that had run down the length of his shirt.

I knelt down beside him and told him not to move and especially not to move his right arm. I grabbed the trauma scissors and quickly cut his shirt off of him. At this time, Jim had left the room and went out to the ambulance to get the MAST pants. As I looked at his entrance wound I noticed that he was a little short of breath. I pulled him away from the back of the couch so I could see his back. As I removed what was left of his shirt, I immediately saw an exit wound. The deputy sheriff noticed that the bullet had gone through the couch and he found where it had lodged in the knotty pine wall.

Just as I was ready to put an occlusive dressing on either side of his right thorax, the officer asks the patient the whereabouts of the gun. Then without saying a word—and without any warning—the patient makes a sudden and extremely fast lunge to the floor. In an instant his hands are under the scattered newspapers. Without hesitation I grab at his hands because I know instinctively that he is going for his gun.

In a millisecond I'm thinking, I might get shot right here and right now! I can't believe this; I might just get myself killed in the next five seconds. It was almost like a dream. It seemed so surreal. I know things were happening in milliseconds and yet it seemed in a way that everything was happening in slow motion. As I looked at the end of his forearms, which were covered with newspapers, I was trying to find his hands and the gun I know he was reaching for. If I get to his hands before he gets to the gun, fine. If I happen to get to the gun before he does, fine. If he gets control of the gun before I can reach his hands, big trouble.

As I scramble to the floor with the patient, deputy Chandler literally did a dive over the couch and knocked us both into the coffee table; knocking it over. The patient gained control of the gun and had it in his right hand. I had his right wrist in a death grip with my left hand and the pistol barrel in my right hand. The deputy sheriff quickly gained hold of the patient's right arm and had control of his general movements.

While this was happening, my partner was just walking back into the room with the MAST pants. He told me later that when he saw this, he was too far away to be of any assistance and close enough to get shot. So Jim just did about the only thing he could do; and that was a big 180, and got the hell out of the way. In retrospect I can't say that I blamed him in the least.

"Drop it! Drop the gun! Just drop it!" I screamed. He loosened his grip, and I quickly slid the gun on the floor where the deputy sheriff quickly gained control of the loaded weapon that was in a semi-automatic mode.

As I look back on that call, I don't know whether or not our patient would have tried to kill either the Deputy Sheriff or myself. He obviously didn't care much for himself. Therefore my thinking was that he probably had less concern for the life or safety of anyone else.

As luck would have it, our patient's only injury was a "through and through" wound to his right lung. Once we got him to the hospital, and the emergency room staff figured out the extent of his injury, they had him patched up in no time. They inserted a chest tube to re-inflate his lung and admitted him to one of the medical floors. What it meant at the time was that he really lucked out.

Chapter 8
IT'S NOT ABOUT THE "N" WORD

At the time of this publication, I am a 58-year-old white male who is gainfully employed as a professional paramedic. For the record, I am a part-time dealer at a local Indian casino, hold an elected public office as a Township trustee, and officiate high school sports. In the recent past, I have been a successful small business owner, school board member and a high school football coach.

I have been and am presently married. My wife, Peggy and I have a daughter and two sons who are now grown and out of the house. I say all of this because what a person, (me in this case) thinks of other people is directly related to a specific point of view. From the first chapter, you have gotten a sense of how I was raised and what was expected of me on a daily basis.

Anyway, I grew up pretty much in an all-white environment. Our high school student population was no more than 350, and within that population were kids from three or four black families. As I recall, there never seemed to be any problems as far as discrimination was concerned. In fact, my African-American schoolmates were generally quite popular. In high school, one of my closest friends, Fred was classified as "Colored," on his birth certificate.

Today, we are separated by two time zones but we have remained close over the years. He was the best man in my wedding and to this day, my wife and our three children absolutely adore him. Fred's older brother Ken was one of my EMT colleagues when I was still employed at the local township.

When I started to work for Medic 1, things for me changed. I experienced blunt racism, firsthand. It wasn't from watching a white person mistreat or discriminate against an African American or Hispanic person. What I saw for the first time was how I was looked at and treated by People of Color.

I remember responding to a call in the city of Benton Harbor (which is just over 92% African American) about a woman who complained of a simple headache. That type of call is clearly a non-emergency and we responded without lights or siren. It took my partner and I about eight minutes to reach the house. As we got out of the ambulance and walked up to the porch, a man (who turned out to be the woman's brother) suddenly opened the front door of the house.

"It took you white motherfuckers long enough to get here," he said screaming. "Or ain't you interested in helping niggers like us?"

For me, it was like walking headlong into a brick wall. I just stood there, staring at him, absolutely stunned. I didn't know what to think let alone say. Here I was, just doing my job in a sane, rational manner and I hear this man call me a "white motherfucker." Worse yet, he called himself and his family, the N word.

As I tried to get over my shock, my partner bailed us both out by saying to the effect that we got there as quickly as we could and that a headache, regardless of the color of the patient, was not a life-threatening emergency. We got the patient out of the house and she walked to the ambulance. Since she was an unemployed Medicaid recipient she received her all expenses paid, taxpayer-sponsored ride to the local hospital.

Another time I experienced racism, was when I responded to a stabbing at a bar that served predominately African-American clients. I walked in having an unzipped hooded sweatshirt on over my uniform shirt. The hood was down so my head and face could be easily seen.

The woman (who turned out to be the bartender) came up behind me and said, "You're not welcome here!"

I quickly spun around and was ready to get into someone's face. As she saw my uniform and trauma box, she immediately saw her error and quickly retreated back behind the bar. She didn't say another word and consequently no apology was forthcoming.

During my long and storied tenure at Medic 1, there have been dozens of times where African Americans have questioned my professional integrity. It usually comes at me personally by saying that if they were white I would have been at their home much sooner. To make matters worse, when serving white patients, I get backlash about my professionalism in serving them.

One time I was running a call out in Benton Township, which is a large township that surrounds Benton harbor on three sides. Benton Township is fairly evenly divided between the number of people who are either African American and white. I don't recall the particular type of call, but as we arrived and got into the house I received this greeting:

"Were you too busy helping those n***** in the city to help us, or what?"

By the time I heard that I had gained my "sea legs" and I was quick to respond by telling this particular idiot that how fast we got anywhere or to anybody is based solely on availability of the ambulance and severity of the call. Unfortunately, since he had the I.Q. of a short stack of pancakes, I'm fairly certain that quick explanation was well over his head.

Over the years I have from time to time, wondered just what to think about all of this grief when it comes to racial strife. I think it's fair to say that I've had some questions as well as statements about all of this. I've come to the conclusion that it's not about the N word; it's about the S word—Stupid. Let's face at least one indisputable fact. Anybody who dislikes or hates anyone just solely on the basis of skin color is simply stupid. It's really just as simple as that.

But speaking of "stupid"...that leads to my first question. How—in today's age of the Internet, the global economy and the ever-increasing age of high technology in which we live—can somebody be too stupid to read a comic book? How does that happen?

I see a huge number of people who really and truly can't possibly use their heads for anything other than a hat rack. The conclusion: The problem is that a person with a limited vocabulary and self-inflicted substandard level of educationally based intellect or at the very least a sub-par level of common sense will usually say and always think that it's not about them. It's about you (or me in this case).

To the person I'm dealing with, it's about how and why I think and feel about that individual that's the problem or concern. In other words, it's not about the patient, family member or witness being just plainly stupid or at the least, profoundly ignorant. It's about how and why I, as an intellectual person using critical thinking, see this person as I do. That particular person invariably will not see him or herself as uneducated or woefully under-educated. Instead, I am of course, a bigot or a racist. At least that's what I'm told from time to time.

When I get dispatched to the scene of an accident or an illness, I choose to minimize someone's opinion. It's not because their skin color may be different than mine, it's because they are that "S" word, and therefore offer nothing useful to the task at hand.

Before we go any further, let's examine precisely what these "giants of intellect" propose to be talking about, and accusing myself and others in EMS of being. The two terms that I seem to hear the most are the words bigot or racist. Webster defines bigot as: *a person who holds blindly and intolerantly to a particular creed or opinion.*

The definition of a racist seems to come closer to the mark. Webster says that a racist (or racialism) is: *a doctrine or teaching, without scientific support, that claims to find racial differences in character, intelligence that asserts the superiority of one race over others.* To some whose emergency calls I answer, I must be akin to a swastika wearing, goose-stepping, Aryan racist. Of course nothing could be further from the truth.

Another conclusion to the question of how an adult in today's world would allow themselves to grow up too stupid to read a comic book is the lack of a basic education of morality, pride in yourself, humility toward others and common manners that were taught by word and example of loving parents. If a dysfunctional family unit is coupled with a woeful or at the least a substandard public school system the results will be kids growing into adulthood unable to grasp the minimums of activities of daily living, let alone find and correctly fill out a job application form.

The place that I work most of the time is in central Berrien County, which is the extreme southwest corner of Michigan. There are primarily four major cities in the county, two of which are within my service area. The first is St. Joseph and the other is Benton Harbor. St. Joseph is mainly an all-white community that is known predominantly for its affluence. It does have areas that are described as under-class or working poor, but it's basically a fairly well to do community.

The 2010 census stated that Benton Harbor had a population of 10,038 residents, down 10.2% from the 2000 census. Of those who still reside within the city limits, 89.2% are African American and 7.0% are white. It is known first and foremost for being an impoverished town with 48.1% of its residents living at or below the poverty level. The average median income for the state of Michigan is $45,255. The median income for this city's residents as of 2009 was $16,267.

That sum is down from the turn of the century level of $17,491. The once great and proud city has all of the social ills that are consistent with that ubiquitous notoriety.

A river divides the two cities, which used to be called the "twin cities." I assure you there is very little reason to call them the "twin cities" anymore. St. Joseph has a school system that has a reputation of academic excellence, modern campuses and a high degree of parental involvement. Regrettably, Benton Harbor has very little of any of that.

To me, the school system is the heartbeat or the nerve center of any community. If you have seen communities without schools because of consolidation, you've seen communities that have lost a piece of their individual identity. The school system is supposed to be the place where the basis of educating children and young adults (in concert with good parenting) and providing them with the tools to be honest, productive adults takes place. The Benton Harbor school system has failed to educate its students in every way to a degree that spells disaster for kids going out into the world looking for gainful employment or are preparing them to excel at the places of higher education.

Now I didn't say that the Benton Harbor school system is particularly at fault for their educational failures. They are not. The central problem has nothing to do with dilapidated buildings or old computers or whatever. It's fair to say that those particular things don't help in matters of poor education, but it's not even close to the core problem. The overriding problem hasn't a thing to do with the way people are treated racially either. Everybody knows what it is, but doesn't dare say.

The reason is because too many kids in the Benton Harbor school system can't begin to learn let alone excel in the classroom because of their family life. Let me tell you what I have seen. I distinctly remember sitting in my ambulance at a stoplight across from Benton Harbor High School. School had just been dismissed for the day and I didn't notice one student carrying a book (this was the days before book bags). It became obvious to me that nobody was assigning, doing or at the least, taking homework.

As I go into some of these houses, it's nothing short of chaos.

There is no "dinner hour" and the so-called parents are hardly concerned with the whereabouts of their kids, let alone if they are doing homework or are doing well in school. There seems to be no family privacy or any kind of ordered structure. Neighborhood people enter into and leave a family home like it's the local Quick-Mart. I couldn't imagine sitting in my house and look up and see someone in my house that wasn't invited, asked, or needed in my home.

As I go into some of the houses of these students, it's not uncommon to get a call at 2 a.m. and walk into the house and see a TV on and kids sleeping on a broken-down couch. I usually have to step over kids sleeping on the floor to get to the pregnant teenager who is in the kitchen waiting for her ride to the hospital. To top it all off, the mother is sitting there without a man in the house—let alone a husband or father figure.

It's not that bad all of the time…it's that bad, far too often. So the question is: How can any kid of any color be expected to be able to learn and be successful in the classroom with a home environment such as that? The answer is, you can't expect a kid to be successful, even in the best of school systems, or the best of classrooms' with a home life such as that. No amount of money is going to fix that, because money isn't the problem. If it were, it would be incredibly easy to correct.

The lack of a consistent nuclear family is the basic problem. I know there are always exceptions to each rule, so spare me the whining and bitching. In our collective conscious and in our heart of hearts we all know it's true. The biggest detriment to a kid's life is not having a father, especially for a boy. The fact of the matter is that far too many women are willing to get pregnant by design, or are unwilling to use or have their partner's use birth control devices for any one of several reasons, or they are just plain ignorant of the facts of life.

I guess they don't know of the long odds of making anything of themselves by bringing unplanned children into a world where they are woefully ill suited to raise in a home where kids are unable to thrive. For me, to see this hopeless situation the many hundreds of times over the more than thirty-five years I've worked at Medic1, is truly disheartening.

With an average income of barely a third of the State's average and in dire need of financial assistance and sustenance, I could only imagine what it must be like, being forever dependent on the government for your meager income, health care, home, utilities, food, and your very own kids' everyday support. The only thing worse is the male population that refuses to support their women, children, and community. Real men don't do that. Real men take responsibility for the financial as well as the emotional and moral support of their families. Somehow it became okay to sweet talk a woman, leave your DNA behind and exit out the back door. Hurricane Katrina never left as much social wreckage behind as that kind of behavior. It's really too bad because Uncle Sam makes for a very poor surrogate father.

The second question is this. Where did this sense of entitlement come from? How did it become okay to make a living by going to the local Department of Social Services and sign up for every freebie under the sun? How did it become okay to then visit your mailbox once a month and cash a welfare check? At what time did it become okay to not at least attempt to earn your own way through life? Finally, at what time did it not become okay to be a positive role model for your children?

How do I know these things? I ask the people I see, medically treat, and otherwise interface with. I ask people about their insurance plan or coverage after medical treatment is concluded and during our transportation time to the local hospital. I ask them whether they are employed, and if so, where. And if they are not employed, I ask them why they are not.

I know a woman who works for the local Department of Social Services. She told me that she has about 300 clients that she serves. She also told me that at least seventy-five percent of the people she sees are just trying in one way or another to scam and cheat the system. I knew the percentage was high, but I was stunned when she told me just how high it actually was. In retrospect, it's not really that surprising. There have been hundreds of people who say and claim to be "disabled" because of the "bad back" syndrome. Of course, that's after I pick them up at a local basketball court for an ankle sprain or they were just stabbed after getting into a bar fight.

Let's not forget the people who are unemployable because of

"substance abuse" issues. What a crock. These aren't people with weaknesses. They are just weak-minded people who usually make it a habit of making poor decisions. My conclusion is that these people play and prey upon the magnanimity and generosity of other people. There is no real concern of making, or at least attempting to make a decision that would show some initiative of obtaining gainful employment or giving a hoot about anything that concerns anyone other than themselves. Astonishingly, many of these same people don't even care about their own well-being.

The reason for that is also remarkably simple, well known, but never spoken. The reason is that if they don't or won't take care of themselves or their families, the tax-paying public will. There seems to be no sense of pride, self worth, goals or any plan of action of any kind. It's just status quo. I see it as a wasted life that is hopelessly meaningless. Like I said before, it's really, really disheartening.

I also know that no racial group has cornered the market on being a bunch of slugs and a drag on society. The fact is however, I work as a paramedic in a predominantly poor black community that is primarily surrounded by several white rural or suburban communities. The social stresses that are mainly in the black community are born from poor family structure, little to no work ethic and a lack or appreciation of a top-notch education.

(I have very little doubt that if I were employed in a predominantly poor white community where there was a palpable absence of a father figure in the house, a no-reason-to-work attitude and pervasive ignorance, those same social stresses would present themselves in exactly the same manner.)

On top of not having positive role models in their personal lives, there seems not to be any positive national role models. With the likes of Jesse Jackson, Al Sharpton and Louis Farrakhan telling their constituents how "put upon" they are by the white man, who can blame them? They tell people that someone else owes them something. They say that although lawful slavery was ended in the 1860s, that somehow they, as descendants of those slaves, are owed money and or property or whatever, for an injustice they did not themselves incur.

What's more, other people who hadn't even been born at the time of slavery and were of course, never slave owners, owe them this.

They tell people they are cheated out of the American dream or are mistreated simply because they are victims of blatant racism. What a joke! The problem is it's not funny. It's a tragedy that's played out everyday across our great nation.

Black leaders who I just mentioned—who espouse looking 50, 100 or 150 years back in time and then telling the African-Americans in this country that they can't be successful without a government handout, or are incompetent socially, morally or financially— are nothing short of traitors to their race.

They fly on their privately-owned or chartered jets all over this country, and every country in the world that has electricity in most places, to denigrate and vilify other people for the misfortune that some have because of the choices that the so called "unfortunate ones" make in the first place. Whereas, they ought to be telling those same people to stop looking back to things you cannot change, get your act together today, and look toward a brighter, self-sustaining tomorrow with a solid plan of action. In short, find a reason to get out of bed, each and every morning.

Furthermore, I would even venture to say that even though we all find the very thought of slavery repugnant, that the descendants of those very same slaves are blessed because they today are living in America. Because Africans were sold and bought into slavery, the descendants of those same slaves that currently live in this country and are United States citizens, enjoy every opportunity to obtain a greater education, multiple job opportunities and a quality of life that still, more than ever, eludes most Africans today.

As for me, my ancestors fled many parts of an impoverished Europe, to cross a vast ocean, and sailed into an uncertain future in the hopes to find a better life. I understand they weren't ripped from their homelands and sold into a cruel and crushing life of slavery, as were the ancestors of many African-Americans. But the point is this: "we", who call ourselves Americans; "we", of every stripe, color and creed who lawfully reside and are called United States citizens are blessed to live here, still, the best country on the planet.

I have another question. Why are people like Dr. Ben Carson, Condoleezza Rice, Clarence Thomas, J.C. Watts, Oprah Winfrey, Colin Powell and the late greats like Arthur Ashe and Reggie White never, or at best, seldom held up as positive role models? These are the types of people who would greatly benefit young people of every color and especially young and adolescent African-Americans.

The reason is remarkably simple. The aforementioned people made it pretty much on their own. They didn't need a government program to excel or succeed. They didn't listen to the people who said they were too under-privileged to make it without the help of an unending government handout. They did it the old fashioned way. They earned it.

I'm sure the way each of them succeeded is a little different, but you can bet that each of them worked their butts off to make their dreams a reality. With that kind of self-motivation, work ethic and focus, most of us have a better than an even chance of being successful at anything that is remotely reasonable.

Of course that puts people like Jackson, Sharpton, Farrakhan and their ilk, right out of business. Those people have a financial investment in the perpetual misery or the perceived misery of others. I can tell you this; people like my best friend Fred, and others just like him regard themselves as fiercely independent and self-sustaining at every level. They don't need or want anyone speaking for them other than themselves. The "Fred's" of this country are more than willing and are readily able to fight their own battles that life brings each of us from time to time.

I have seen first hand African-American families and have been in their homes where Dad is and has always been present. There is pride, individual respect, family unity and order, and an emphasis for kids to excel in school. It's impressive to witness. It's a place where you "feel" how proud people can be when they can say that they and only they have earned this or that. They are quick to point out that nobody gave them anything.

They are insistent that they don't want or expect something for nothing, just a fair shot at their attempt to attain a particular goal. It's a way of living, no matter the color of your skin, which has a high degree of integrity that deserves and demands respect. As odd as it may seem, as a paramedic, I don't get called to those houses very often. Then again, over the years I've been in some houses more times than I've been in some neighborhoods.

I have seen over the years, literally thousands of times, people calling the local EMS provider to go to the hospital, by ambulance, for something as mundane as a headache or a scrape on the elbow. Think about that for a minute. Can anyone who values a dollar explain to me what kind of mentality it takes for a person who wants to go to a hospital for a simple headache or a minor scrape to the elbow? And then wants or expects to go to that same hospital by an ambulance?

It's a total misuse of resources and a colossal waste of taxpayer dollars. What kind of person does that? Any self-respecting person would not want to be a burden or would be ashamed and deeply embarrassed to do such a thing.

I don't mean to be a harsh, but let's face it. You could buy a two-dollar box of Band-Aids or a bottle of generic aspirin, Tylenol or Ibuprophen and take them as prescribed, or you could incur the costs of several hundred taxpayer dollars. As for the answer, what kind of person calls an ambulance for a regular, mundane headache? It's easy and we all know. And no, it's not a person who doesn't own or have access to a car or other transportation. If that were the reason then those people wouldn't be able to get themselves back home (and they always find a way home).

It's the kind of person who doesn't work and thinks someone else owes them a living. And that's the key. For too many people, there is no personal cost. They have Medicaid or no insurance at all. For them, it's as simple as picking up a phone and having someone else take care of the most minor of medical problems.

When I have to respond to a call such as that, and when I arrive, I'm already aggravated. Admittedly, I walk in with a chip on my shoulder. Sometimes I don't handle it as well as I should. I'll be the first to say that I am not totally guiltless when getting into it with someone over a racial issue or actually, more to the point of a social responsibility issue.

***

During one of our usual twenty-four hour shifts, we had been getting kicked around all day by just running one ambulance call after another. It was just one of those days where it seemed like everybody in the city needed an ambulance for one thing or another. Randy and I had handled everything from the, "Help me, I've fallen and I can't get up" call, to heart attacks, to multiple patient car accidents, to the many area nursing homes that have the old fossils who are 89 years old and trying really hard not to reach 90.

I don't remember exactly but we were on our seventeenth or eighteenth ambulance call when at about 2 a.m. we got a call to a house where someone in their mid-twenties reportedly was having a seizure. We hadn't had time to eat since before noon and hadn't been to sleep at all. Nonetheless, we were still going strong and we are now into our 19th hour of non-stop work.

It's been my experience that when someone between the ages of 20 and 50 is having a seizure, it's because they are out of medicine and haven't taken it upon themselves to get it refilled or they are seizure patients who are heavily intoxicated. At any rate, again someone hasn't made the best of decisions and now his or her bad choices in life are involving me and I'm irritated about it ... again.

We arrived at our destination and got out of the ambulance to hear a whole bunch of yelling, arguing, screaming, cussing and just a lot of chaos. So we walked up to the door and then announced that the paramedics are here.

Just as soon as Randy got those words out of his mouth, a female voice says, "Get yo' white asses in here!"

I instantly thought to myself, "Oh man, not this crap again". When I looked at Randy and from the expression on his face, I knew he had the exact same thought as I did.

We entered the house to see one man and six women. The call for the ambulance was for a woman who was lying on the floor. So I asked what had happened to the woman on the floor to the one woman who appeared to be the least intoxicated. She was being generally helpful when another woman started asking us questions about why it took us so long to get there. At first we just ignored her, but she was persistent as well as obnoxious. So my good friend and then partner, Randy Garnett, is attempting in vain to explain that sometimes seconds seem like minutes and minutes seem like hours, and that it really didn't take very long at all to arrive.

While he is doing that, I had my back to them and I'm kneeling on the floor next to the "patient". The woman that Randy is now arguing with is getting more irritated and louder by the minute, to the point of being really irrational and highly confrontational. It's now to the point where he has to push her away so she doesn't strike either one of us.

As I try to hear and record a blood pressure, I can't hear anything through my stethoscope except her yelling and Randy doing his best to calm her down. Finally, I had had enough.

I quickly got to my feet, spun around and yelled to her to "shut the hell up!" I then turned to Randy and said, "Don't say another damn thing to her! She's obviously dumber than dirt!"

She then comes at me and Randy grabs her by the face and pushes her away yet again. Not to be deterred, she screams at me and says, "If she'd be white, she'd be at the hospital by now!" That was the last straw.

I just blew a gasket and screamed back at her and said, "You know, you're right! If she was white, she'd be at the hospital (as I snapped my fingers an inch from her nose), that fast!"

Of course I said that for her benefit and I immediately turned my back to her just to infuriate her all the more. I then knelt down to the woman on the floor (who by the way was faking this whole seizure episode) to take the blood pressure cuff off of her arm.

As I was kneeling I could see the woman I had just given the insult to, coming at me. I thought nothing of it because Randy "had my back" and after all, I'm thinking she isn't a linebacker for the Chicago Bears or anything such as that. She's just an averaged sized woman who happens to be ignorant, mouthy, obnoxious and really, really drunk.

Randy attempts to push her away like he did six or eight times before when she leans back and delivers a roundhouse punch and puts it right square on his jaw. Of course I didn't find that out until later. At the time that happened, the only thing I knew for sure was that Randy was falling backwards over me and he was landing right on top of the woman who was pretending to be unconscious. At that instant I scrambled to my feet as fast as I could, ready to get into the fight that I thought was quickly coming upon us.

As I'm getting to my feet, the woman on the floor miraculously is awakened to someone landing full force on top of her. Now she is as mad as all hell and starts trying to get to her feet and beat on Randy, all at the same time. Meanwhile Randy is trying not to get punched again and grabs the walkie-talkie that he is carrying and starts screaming for dispatch to send the police. By this time, the two women that all of this involved, are running out of the house so they aren't taken to jail when the police arrive.

During this whole fiasco, the only guy in the house never said a word to us and never raised a finger to help or hinder. He wasn't any trouble at all and really didn't seem to be concerned at all to what was just going on. He just sat on the couch behind their coffee table, downing shots of whiskey and watching the show.

At the time, none of it seemed very funny at all. But as time goes on, you gain a different perspective on certain events. The number-one thing is that I shouldn't have lost my temper as I did. The second thing is that we should have called for the police when the first argument started. Honestly speaking, we mostly look back on it as a really funny event. It's been at least ten years since that particular call and I still haven't bought Randy dinner for taking that punch on the jaw for me.

***

In yet another time where I got a bunch of unwarranted grief for not arriving at a scene quickly enough because the person hurt in the car accident was African-American (as if we would know that prior to our arrival), was during a call, where we responded to a two car, head-on accident. After arriving on the scene of the collision, we asked if any of the nearly two-dozen onlookers knew what happened. Several said that they heard the impact, but none had actually seen the collision.

The injured driver of the one car complained of neck and back pain. He also said his legs "felt numb and heavy." I told him that I understood that he had back pain but I had to check him thoroughly before we would be removing him from his car. I told him that if he has too much pain (in his back in this case), that it could mask other injuries that he might have sustained. He understood.

Unfortunately, not everybody was appreciative of the time it took to properly care for the hurt man. There was one loud mouth in the crowd who was just sure that we were wasting time by not getting this person to the hospital in what he thought was a timely fashion. After further examination I had ascertained that my patient also had a broken left forearm, clavicle and possible rib fractures. I knew the time needed for this particular extrication from the car would be lengthy.

I recorded a full set of vital signs and then started an IV and administered oxygen before applying the first splint to the patient. I then retreated back to the ambulance to retrieve the needed equipment for the careful removal of our patient from his wrecked car.

As my partner and I were gathering our equipment, I started to hear the "cat calls" referencing the time taken because our patient happened to be African American. Again, there were few things in life that irritate me more than some moron playing the Race card who doesn't have the foggiest notion on what they are seeing, much less talking about.

As I got back to the side of my patient, I knew he was hearing this dumb ass in the sizeable crowd continue to chastise me and my partner. I told my patient not to worry about what was being said. I told him that the loud mouth in the crowd didn't have a clue as to what we were doing or why and reiterated that we were taking our time as to not make any mistakes that may cause him to be in a wheel chair for the rest of his life. To say the least, he was extremely grateful for our professional treatment. We had our splints, KED board and backboard all piled on top of our cot.

I was going back and forth between the cot and the car when that same meathead said, "Move your ass, you white bastard!"

I snapped back at him as I grabbed the KED board and held it out to him and shouted, "Hey wise guy, do you want me to step back so you can put this thing on?"

He retorts, "I want you to do your job, mother fucker!"

I responded by yelling back to him, "Step back asshole and I'll do my job!"

Some of the people in the crowd stepped up by getting this idiot out of my face. They too, were less than kind and considerate to this dumb ass while they told him to keep quiet, and to let us do our jobs.

The people in the large crowd showed us great support. In fact, I enlisted the help of two guys to assist us with the final removal of our patient out of his car.

Through it all and over the years, I have never mistreated anyone who has needed my services. However, I do from time to time challenge people who use me as a convenient taxi. I have never once given a different course of treatment because of the color of someone's skin. That simply would not happen. In all honesty, I have never seen malpractice or maltreatment of a patient by any EMS worker at Medic 1 or any other ambulance service, for that matter on the basis of skin color.

Furthermore, it's been my experience that I have never observed a nurse or doctor anywhere mistreating anyone because they didn't like the pigment of their skin. Good people from all races and walks of life wouldn't for a minute allow it or sit still for it. I believe that people who are either ill or injured often need EMS and to that end, the color of someone's skin is totally irrelevant. My only concern is whether you are in dire need, serious need, in need of transportation only or are just wasting my time. The answers to those questions will directly dictate how I choose to interact with those who I see. For me, it's really just that simple. Racism in EMS? I don't believe it exists. It may have occurred in the distant past, but not where I work and not today.

Chapter 9
COLONELS AND CORPORALS

Paramedics— and to a lesser degree emergency medical technicians (EMT's)—work on an established set of protocols that cover just about any kind of traumatic or medical emergency. It's the Project Medical Director (PMD) who is ultimately responsible and oversees all EMS activity in a given county. The PMD is responsible for basically everyone who is licensed to come to the aid of someone else. To that end, they literally put their medical licenses on the line each time a paramedic opens a drug box or interprets an EKG rhythm. So it's very understandable that they may be somewhat concerned about paramedics doing the right thing for the right reason. Nobody has any legitimate argument with that.

A great or even a good paramedic has no problem understanding that we are indeed not doctors and don't pretend to be. That's why I think that paramedics who are new to the business, inexperienced, or are just unsure of how to do one thing or another, use protocols as an "etched in granite" way of treating their patients.

Actually, this will work well about 98% of the time. However, if you continually rely on a follow-the-numbers way of treating patients, you will eventually get stuck and it usually means that you will not be treating your patient as well as possible to alleviate their pain or discomfort. In the worst-case scenario, it may mean big trouble for the outcome of your patient.

However, there are times where protocols don't fit the particular emergency or the particular patient you are treating. For that reason, it's my belief that protocols are best used as a general guide on how patients should be treated.

Too often there are too many exceptions to all of these rules. Great and even good to average emergency room doctors understand that. They know all too well that the phrase "practicing medicine" means that diagnosing and treating patients is as much as an art form as it is a science. They also know that once in a while paramedics can treat two similar patients with the same exact complaint and end up with two very different patient outcomes. It just happens that way.

Conversely, the same is true with doctors. A paramedic could treat a patient and depending on how he treats that particular patient and what happened, he may get two very different reactions from two different doctors.

Most of the time, a paramedic will give a brief report to the doctor as to how the patient presented, his general complaint, vital signs, the patients initial symptoms and of course, what invasive procedures you performed. Equally important is how the patient reacted to the therapy that was given and how their condition has changed.

Once in a while, the patient will have an extended medical history that may determine a certain course of treatment or the treatment itself may be more protracted than usual. Either of these incidents will need to be explained to the doctor and or the attending nurse. It's not unusual for this to happen. How some doctors react are at times, more than a little unusual.

There are those doctors who treat us with the respect we have earned through thousands of hours of study and years of experience. Many times those doctors were once paramedics themselves and truly understand the plight paramedics and EMT's face when they are fighting the good fight on behalf of their critically ill or injured patient or patients.

They understand the chaos that has to be quickly sorted out by EMS professionals. They know how difficult it is to interact and obtain pertinent information from family and friends of those who are stricken. They know how it is to be in the eye of the hurricane. When everyone is losing their composure around them, the attending paramedic must be the one who remains resolute and totally focused on the task at hand.

In those chaotic and challenging times, the professional paramedic must incorporate the help of others to give the patient the best chance of a favorable outcome. That often means getting ordinary citizens and many times family members to help in the emergency. Sometimes that means getting your patient's medicine, moving furniture (to make room for treatment or for getting the ambulance cot to where it needs to be), or getting another family member under control. Sometimes it means just holding an IV bag. The point is this, if you make people around you part of the solution, they won't be part of the problem.

Perhaps the most important thing is leadership. All of the truly great paramedics that I have been fortunate to know over the years had superior leadership skills and ability. It's been my experience over the years, that if you make decisive decisions with confidence and experience, all others will follow. All of the aforementioned obstacles are everyday occurrences in the profession of EMS. The truly great hospital based surgeons and practitioners want to know what EMS personnel have to say about the patient they are delivering to them. To them, we are the "start of the story".

At the other end of the spectrum are those doctors who think paramedics are just dumb ambulance drivers deserving of no respect. They don't understand the essential and often times the critical role that EMS plays (other than a simple transportation service). They don't understand, let alone appreciate, the wide variety of challenges (both big and small) that awaits the professional as well as the volunteer EMS workers on every emergency call. They don't know our capabilities, respect our knowledge, or acknowledge our experience. Some doctors don't even know the difference between basic and advanced life support ambulances.

As they look down their noses at us, they actually think we are all the same. I think the worst thing with these few doctors, is that they don't want to hear anything that you may have to say about the patient that you are delivering to them. The only thing they want to know is: What happened to them? Were they in a car wreck? Did they fall off a ladder? Do they have chest pain?

After that, they have the, "I'll figure it out for myself" attitude. To that end, I have absolutely no respect at all for those types of doctors. (Luckily, those types are fewer and fewer all of the time.) Furthermore, I don't have a single problem telling them as much. I learned a long time ago that respect is a two-way street and I always give as well as I get.

Of the many hospitals that we deliver patients to, one is a small community hospital in Watervliet. The emergency department by most standards is small with less than a dozen beds. It is served by a group of doctors who work a few shifts there and then rotate out to other bigger hospitals. One of the doctors is a really cool guy by the name of Shawn Michaels or I should say Colonel Shawn Michaels. He retired from the U.S. Army Reserves as a full bird colonel and was a deputy Project Medical Director (PMD) that represented Watervliet Community Hospital (WCH) to the local county medical control board. As a point of well-deserved personal pride he served two tours of duty in Iraq.

Whenever I delivered a patient to that small emergency room, I would always hope that he would be working. I always found him to be interesting to converse with. His view on the United States military, Middle East politics and so forth would be topics of conversation that I would thoroughly enjoy. He told me that if he had gone back to the "arena" for another tour, he could have gotten his star.

For me, that was a real head-turner. I found it incredible that he could have been a brigadier general, if he had so chosen. After all, how many military Generals does an ordinary guy like me have for a friend?

After I did my double take at this revelation, I said to him, "You're going to go back, aren't you?"

He looked up at me from the patient chart he was writing on and chuckled. "No, no, I'm done with all of that. Two times over there is enough", was his answer.

Dr. Michaels had a real ease about him. He always seemed relaxed, levelheaded and even-tempered. If there is or was a problem or even a question on how a paramedic treated a particular patient it would get worked out to everyone's satisfaction. You could always see in Dr. Michaels the military discipline and the quiet confidence that brings that type of behavior. There was never any yelling, screaming, or threatening with him for any reason. Inside the emergency room he was unflappable. I would guess that after what he had seen while serving in the military, everything else is somewhat anticlimactic.

At any rate, he is one heck of a doctor as well as a fine and admirable man. All of the paramedics and EMT's at Medic 1 really appreciated Dr. Michaels as the deputy PMD and I know he enjoyed immense respect from all of my colleagues. Before he arrived to his position at the hospital, there were several paramedics from Medic 1 who had problems with the lack of professionalism from some of the nursing staff. He heard all of the complaints, and got it all straightened out. Unfortunately, he later had to resign his position because of his ongoing commitment to the United States military.

The guy who took his place was a real piece of work. Dr. Dipstick (not his real name but his real attitude). He started off by throwing his weight around and trying to reinvent the EMS wheel. He came from a different system where ambulances operated under a very tight medical control. In our particular county, and in our particular system, the paramedics enjoyed a little bit more autonomy than what he was accustomed to or otherwise comfortable with.

The first day that I knew Dr. Dipstick was on the planet, was on a late September day when I had an ambulance call at a local adult assisted-living facility in Baroda, MI. My partner Anthony Pantaleo and I responded to the facility to take care of an elderly woman who had apparently suffered a stroke. Although she was not acutely ill, she was found to be generally in poor health and had a history of several previous strokes. The only thing that was immediately notice-able was that she had facial droop to one side and slurred speech. The caregivers stated that her impaired speech was a new physical finding.

When we began our assessment, we found an 83-year-old lady who was breathing easy and whose vital signs were all within normal limits. She was alert and oriented and could make her own medical decisions. She was also a long ago retired nurse at the Watervliet Community Hospital and also the house supervisor at that particular hospital. That meant she had been in charge of the entire nursing staff at the hospital when she was on duty.

When we arrived at the assisted living center, her son was already at his mother's side. As unbelievable as it may sound, the staff at the facility stated they hadn't seen her in perhaps as much as sixteen hours! Up to this point the call had been pretty mundane. Instead of going to the local hospital, which was about eight miles away, our patient insisted in going to the Watervliet hospital, which was more than twenty miles away.

Since she was not a candidate for thrombolytic treatment (to break up a blood clot that may be causing her stroke), Anthony and I saw no reason whatsoever as to why we could not accommodate her wishes. On top of that, her doctor was from Watervliet and her son was insistent that we take his mom to "her hospital."

Anthony and I looked at each other and he said, "I guess we're going to Watervliet."

I looked back at him and shrugged my shoulders and said, "I have no problem with that."

We placed her on our ambulance cot and administered two liters per minute of oxygen via a nasal cannula. We saw no good reason to start an IV on her, so we started on our way to the hospital of her wishes.

We were perhaps twenty minutes into our twenty-five minute trip to the hospital when I decided to call Watervliet to advise them that they would soon be receiving a patient who had suffered a stroke. I told the nurse who had answered my call, that we had just given her a little oxygen and she could expect us to arrive in about four to five minutes. After hearing my brief summation, the nurse quickly demanded that I start an IV on our patient.

Since paramedics don't take orders directly from nurses and since I disagreed with her request, I chose to not start the IV. In my professional opinion there was no medical reason she needed an IV in the pre-hospital setting. The truth is, it would have been just a courtesy to the hospital staff. Well a courtesy is just that, a courtesy. Frankly speaking, at the time I just didn't feel like being benevolent. Besides about half of the time these types of patients are direct hospital admissions and there is no emergency room intervention.

When we arrived, the emergency room was fairly busy. There was a new doctor working whom I had never seen before that day. At a glance he appeared young, no more than five-feet-ten inches tall with a thin build. He reminded me of the comedian Pee Wee Herman, or some little Ivy League School sissy with a stethoscope hanging from his neck. The attending nurse was the same nurse who I had talked with over the phone when I called the hospital about our patient. After I turned the care of the patient over to the nurse and started my paperwork, she noticed that I had not started the IV that she had requested.

Her body language said it all. The look on her face, the stomping around, the little hand gestures and flippant remarks said silently, "I'm really aggravated with that paramedic." So as a result, I did an admittedly poor job in writing out the patient report form and quickly and quietly exited the hospital. It was that I just didn't want to hear a lot of grief from the nurse and even the new doctor. Anthony and I left and went back to our central area located in Benton Harbor.

As we were still a couple of miles from the station our dispatcher called instructing us to call the Watervliet hospital as soon as possible. I thought, *That's just great! I'm going to get called on the carpet from a doctor whom I've never met, for an IV that simply wasn't needed. Isn't there any end to this stupidity? Are the nurses really that lazy that they can't start their own IV's?*

I ignored the request. As we arrived back at the station, I remembered that the Detroit Lions were playing my beloved Green Bay Packers. As usual, Brett Favre was having another stellar performance and I, along with Anthony and two other guys were really enjoying the game.

About ten minutes later, the phone rang, and our dispatcher said over the intercom, "Hey Jim, it's Dr. 'Dipstick', and he wants to talk to you."

"Tell him I'm not here right now!" I yelled back.

A few seconds later, Jason walks out of the dispatch room into our big TV room and says, "C'mon Stine, if I tell him that, he's just going to keep calling us back."

Knowing that the dispatcher is one of those kinds of guys who is really pretty orderly, straight-laced, and honest and generally doesn't like a lot of grief, I looked at him from the couch I was sitting on enjoying the football game and said, "Oh, all right!" I just couldn't believe this new idiot doctor is going to climb all over my ass about an IV that medically means nothing.

I picked up one of our several extensions, pushed the blinking red button and said, "Hello, my I help you?"

The voice on the other end of the phone line said, "This is Dr. Dipstick. Is this the paramedic who just brought Mrs. Smith to the Watervliet hospital?"

"Yes it is. What can I do for you?"

"You can start off by telling me the reason as to why you took Mrs. Smith up here to Watervliet instead of over to Lakeland Hospital which was only eight miles away?"

I couldn't have been more pleasantly surprised not to mention, relieved. Here I thought all of this time that I was going to get reamed out for not starting an IV. I could tell by the tenor of the doctor's voice he was angry about our decision, but I was still relieved it wasn't about that IV.

So in a matter of fact voice, I said, "Sure doc, I'll give you five reasons. First off she was hemodynamically sound. Two, she isn't a candidate for thrombolytic therapy. Three, her doctor is from Watervliet. Four, her son who was on scene, insisted that we take her to Watervliet. And five, and most importantly, that's where she wanted to go. So what's your problem?"

Now Dr. Dipstick was really miffed because I gave him five really sound reasons why he received this patient.

"I'll tell you what my problem is!" he yelled. " Who do you think you are that you can make these kinds of medical decisions without calling medical control?"

At that precise moment, I thought to myself, I always make these kinds of medical decisions. Up to this time I have been doing so for more than twenty-five years. I also thought in that same precise second, Hey, I'm not going to be talked to this way, particularly from some putz that I don't even know. Besides the Green Bay Packers are playing football right this minute.

So I did something that I have regretted for more than two years...I unilaterally discontinued our conversation. At the time I didn't give a damn about my show of disrespect. I figured that if he wanted to talk to me over the phone in that manner, he didn't deserve any respect from me, at all!

In retrospect, that was clearly the wrong thing to do. What I should have done was to cut him off in mid rant and say, "Hold on there, doc. I don't know you and I don't know who you think you are, and by your demeanor, you sure as hell don't know me. So unless you want a real problem on your hands you had best check your tone and calm down!"

That's what I earnestly wished I had done instead of hanging up on him. But my beloved Packers were kicking the stuffing out of the Lions and I didn't want to miss the game on account of this ridiculous doctor and his idiotic concerns.

As a result of my foolish decision, all hell was unleashed in my direction. From what I understand, he called my boss and wanted me immediately suspended. Since the guy who I work for and Dr. Dipstick were having problems on another front, that wasn't going to happen, not to mention there was no merit for any suspension. But the snit the good doctor was having wasn't going to abate for more than two years.

After calling my boss, he called some of his colleagues in the area he was originally from and asked their opinions on what had transpired between the two of us. Since they are probably cut from the same cloth, they said that they wouldn't stand for such insubordination and he should immediately call the PMD and have him remove my practicing privileges at once.

The PMD in our county at the time was a guy by the name of Dr. Robert Kraff. He's a good guy and had a very low key and relaxed way of controlling EMS in our county. He was more of a moderator than a hard-nosed, do it my way or else type of guy. I know that I and the vast majority of the paramedics in this county really appreciated the fact that if you had any reasonable problem with hospital personnel, medical protocols or just had an idea that you thought had some merit on pre-hospital patient care, you could go in and have an informal sit down conversation with him. He was always interested to hear what paramedics had to say about improving or changing the way we deliver care to our patients.

Dr. Kraff and I go back more than twenty-five years and he knows me and my capabilities as a paramedic very well. As a result, I always enjoyed a certain degree of latitude as a paramedic in his system. He also knows my character and integrity as a man. So just because I took this doctor down a couple of notches by not kissing his ass and saying how wrong I was for not taking Mrs. Smith to the closest hospital (because I'm just a dumb ambulance driver), the chances for a suspension of any kind would have been very remote. As a matter of fact, it wasn't even considered.

To top it all off, I happened to see a copy of the letter that Dr. Dipstick wrote to the Michigan Dept. of Public Health (MDPH) the state licensing board and demanded that my paramedic license be revoked. Among other things stated in the letter was that I "posed a danger to the community." On a professional basis, I've never been so chastised, humiliated and deeply insulted. I thought back to all of the literally thousands of people who I have assisted through times of extreme and life threatening needs with my chosen profession.

I thought and reflected on the pain and suffering that I have eased or alleviated and even pondered with great satisfaction the lives that I had managed to save over the more than twenty-five years of dedicated service. I thought about the really great reputation that I have (or had) with all of the doctors and nurses that I interact with on a nearly daily basis. Now all of this may be ruined because of this knuckle-headed doctor who doesn't even know me, let alone know my capabilities. I was just emotionally devastated, not to mention as perhaps as angry at any one individual as I have ever been.

When I saw that letter to the state, I knew from that moment forward, I was going to make this an all out war. From his perspective he probably thought, "By God, I'm going to get my pound of flesh, one way or another out of this bad paramedic". What he didn't know was that I don't cut so easily. If he wanted trouble and controversy, he was going to get plenty. As far as that goes, most veteran paramedics know just how far they can "push the envelope" and that it is certainly an art form. So now it's just a matter of time and for me just a matter of being patient. My singular goal in my professional life from that moment forward was to anger and irritate this arrogant ass just as much as I possibly could. As providence would have it, I wouldn't have to wait long. Little did I know it, but my first salvo was going to be fired over the telephone.

After a few months went by, and many phone calls between Dr. Kraff and ole' Dipstick, Dr. Kraff in an attempt to put this feud to rest and placate Dipsticks' wounded ego, called me and insisted that I do three things. The first was to rewrite Mrs. Smith's medical control form that I wrote out so haphazardly, as an addendum to the original. I was more than happy to do that part of his request.

The second thing was that Dr. Dipstick insisted that I go through the American Heart Association's, Advanced Cardiac Life Support (ACLS) textbook. I was to look through and read the stroke management section. First off and foremost, I already had done that several times over the many years that I had been a practicing paramedic. As part of our job requirement, all of the paramedics must maintain current certification as an ACLS provider.

It's an every two-year re-certification that usually takes about six to eight hours to complete. It includes the latest information and technology on all aspects of treating cardiovascular emergencies, the latest way to do cardiopulmonary resuscitation (CPR), cardiac rhythm recognition, written tests and several practical stations that test your knowledge in advanced airway management, and treating cardiac arrests that happen by circumstances that are numerous to say the least.

Because I already had read the section on pre-hospital stroke management care, I clearly understood those patient's who were candidates for therapy that would dissolve clots in the brain and reverse or at the least, minimize the effects of a stroke and those who would not be viable candidates. It wasn't because I didn't know the difference or was ignorant to Mrs. Smith's medical options. It was precisely because we did know Mrs. Smith's medical options, and it's why we agreed to take her to Watervliet in the first place.

That really irritated me, but because I admired Dr. Kraff and respected him, I again read over the text.

The third thing was to be the toughest and that was to call and talk with Dr. Dipstick about stroke management. After he tried to get me basically fired from my job (after all there isn't a lot of need for paramedics who can't practice), the last thing I wanted to do was to talk with this guy. So I just wouldn't do it. Finally about ninety days or so after the incident—and I'm sure after much additional prodding from Dr. Dipstick—Dr. Kraff called me at my home and basically pleaded with me for the sake of harmony to call this insolent, self-important ass and talk with him.

I argued with Dr. Kraff for more than twenty minutes about this arrogant bastard from Watervliet and how he tried to ruin my professional life. And now, I'm supposed to play nice. As far as I was concerned, the time for that had long passed. Finally Dr. Kraff reminded me of how long we had known each other and how much mutual respect we had for one another and told me that he would consider it a personal favor to him if I would just pick up the phone and talk with Dr. Dipstick. After that, what could I say other than yes?

"I'll do it for you and only you, Dr. Kraff," is exactly what I said. As it turned out, it wasn't to be nearly that easy.

During this whole three to four month time period, there were things going on at the hospital that would affect EMS in Berrien County. Dr. Kraff, our project medical director for more than twenty years, was stepping down. Dr. Royale was replacing him. Dr. Dipstick wanted the job, but the powers that be wouldn't give it to him because he didn't work at the principle hospital where the medical control authority originated. Life would have been miserable with that pinhead in charge, particularly for me.

Anyway Dr. Royale pretty much picked up where Dr. Kraff left off. By this time, Dr. Royale had gotten the full story, my version as well as Dipsticks' rendition. It seemed to me that whoever talked with Dr. Royale last seemed to have his favor. I kept on talking and putting off calling Dipstick, mostly just to irritate him. When I didn't call, he'd raise all kinds of hell and complain to Dr. Royale that I put him off yet again. As I said before, I know how much I can push the envelope and the paper was getting tight.

After trying to dodge talking to Dr. Dipstick, Dr. Royale suggested I call him by a date in early February or lose my privileges to practice. I had obviously stretched it to the breaking point. I waited until late into the night on the day before the final day and I called. I waited until that day mostly just to irritate Dipstick, but also and more importantly, because I was scheduled to work at our central station. Because it's our dispatch center as well, all of the phone calls are recorded. So I called him and wouldn't you know it, I got his recording. Well, I left my very brief message and about two minutes later, he called me back.

I really didn't know how it would go and since I'm still stinging over him calling me a "danger to the community," I'm honestly hoping it doesn't go well at all. Furthermore, I hope he makes a mistake. Whether it comes from a job threat or a medical matter, for me, it doesn't make any difference.

He started off by thanking me for calling him and wanted to know if I had read the required information. Technically I had read the same information several years in a row and I didn't need to read it again. I could have said, "Yes, I read it." But I'm generally an honest guy, and I feel uncomfortable telling any lie. So I told him I had read the same stroke protocols in the past and I know the treatments hadn't changed, so I felt that I didn't need to read something again that I already knew.

He then started in by attempting to give me an oral quiz over the phone. When I first talked to Dr. Royale about my calling Dr. Dipstick, I distinctly remember complaining about the possibility of him giving me some oral quiz while I talked to him. It wasn't the content of his questions that concerned me at all. It was just the fact this egotistical ass would be talking down to me. The idea of that just pissed me off more than I can say. I told Dr. Royale that and I remember him telling me not to worry about that. "Just talk to him about the call", he said.

After a forty-four minute conversation the two of us continue to go back and forth on why I didn't start an IV and take her to the nearest facility. He continued to threaten me with suspension and I keep demanding on what grounds that should happen.

The facts are, the reason you start an IV are three-fold: 1) You want to give your patient fluid (and that can be for several reasons). 2) You want to give your patient an intravenous drug. 3) In case something happens to your patient while you are enroute to the hospital you have a quick access into their circulatory system.

The fact is I wasn't going to give her any fluids or drugs. Further, if she had exhibited any signs or symptoms of distress of any kind, it would not have been an issue. So the likelihood of anything else happening is extremely remote. If the powers that be were concerned of what might happen, nobody would ever leave the hospital after being treated with any malady. Furthermore, I might have to start an IV on everybody who leaves a bar, restaurant or nightclub because they might get into an accident on their way home. The whole thing is utterly ridiculous and borders on sublime idiocy.

JS: "It was so mundane, so routine; I didn't think it was necessary. Yeah, it was a judgment call on my part, but I'm waiting to hear where the patient was compromised because of the lack of this IV lock........."

DD: "That's just one less step we have to do in the emergency room."

JS: "And there you go, it's a courtesy. As far as that patient is concerned, one hundred percent of the paramedics would have taken that patient, in that condition, to Watervliet as requested by that patient and her family. One hundred times out of one hundred times!"

DD: Then the protocols would have been violated............."

JS: "Doc, I just got our protocol book here and you're talking about the altered mental status, is that correct?"

DD: "Right."

JS: "Well it says under management here...and it says in bold print, if your patient is not alert or vital signs are unstable...obtain vascular access. Now this patient that we are in some sort of disagreement over was alert and very stable. So under that particular protocol, I think everything was handled quite appropriately...if that's the protocol that you're talking about?"

DD: "Well that's about as close as we have to a stroke protocol."

It turns out that we really don't have a particular or unique protocol that covers people who suffer strokes. What it does say is how to treat symptoms of a stroke. He then asks me about giving aspirin to someone with a stroke. That caught me a little off-guard because that is about the last thing we would do. The fact is the only time we give aspirin is to patients who we suspect are having heart attacks.

His first mistake was a patient assessment mistake. Now he is clearly making not only a protocol mistake but a mistake in general medicine as far as stroke management is concerned.

I'm pointing out to the good doctor how aspirin isn't in the stroke (or altered mental status) protocol at all. So now it is clear to us that good 'ole Dr. Dipstick doesn't know what he's talking about. But does that little fact slow him down? Well heaven knows, not at all. After all, he's "the doctor".

Now he switches gears. He's starts in by talking about what is in the Advanced Cardiac Life Support textbook. Although it is clearly a learning tool, it doesn't mean that we follow those particular procedures all of the time. So the bottom line is this, he couldn't nail me to the cross via the protocol route, so now he's attempting to do it with a textbook.

Again, he switches gears by talking about hypertension in acute stroke. He insists that we are to give nitroglycerin to reduce the blood pressure. It used to be that way, but we no longer do that because of the risk of non-perfusion to the immediate area around the area of the brain where the stroke occurred.

(When I played this tape recording to Dr. Royale the following day, he actually winced when he heard 'ole Dipstick spout off about how we should be attempting to reduce blood pressure with people afflicted with a stroke. His exact words were, "That's not right. I'll have to talk with him about that.")

He switches gears yet again, and starts hammering me about not taking the patient to the nearest medical facility. He follows that with "You always do what's in the best interest of the patient", routine. What he keeps failing to acknowledge is that overall, Anthony and I did exactly the right thing for the right patient for the right reasons. Although I didn't document it properly, everything turned out exactly how it should have turned out for the patient.

By this time he is reminding me of someone who has their car stuck in the snow. He just keeps throwing the gearshift between forward and reverse, and all the while he is just spinning his wheels.

After listening again and again to the recording of my conversation with Dr. Dipstick, it remains clear to me that he was here to twist me in the wind for not giving him the respect that he thought was due him. Although it was wrong of me to hang up on him while I was talking with him on the phone those many months previous to our latest conversation that I just recorded, it probably remains the only time a lowly paramedic ever disrespected him like that.

His two areas of concern he says were not starting an IV and not taking that particular patient to the nearest hospital were clearly flawed. He says that an ad-hoc committee came to a unanimous conclusion of my guilt in not doing the proper thing or giving the proper care to this patient. In reality, it was this doctor who was undeniably wrong. It is clear to me that it was he who didn't know our protocols of treatment in stroke or altered mental status management. Moreover, I believe that he was bluffing or out right fabricating a story about how this committee came to a "unanimous conclusion" about how wrong I was.

The only thing it would have taken was to have just one member on that ad-hoc committee to open our protocol book, and look into what is supposed to happen. I can hardly believe that didn't or at the least wouldn't have happened at a real meeting. As for the treatment given to our patient is concerned, Anthony and I did everything that was prudent, reasonable and necessary. We carried out our patient's wishes and the wishes of her family. We treated her with expert knowledge and true compassion, respect and dignity.

It is clear to me now, that the good doctor was just trying to bully me and have me beg for my job. Well, that simply was not going to happen. Like most people of his ilk, he is an arrogant ass. Because he is a medical doctor, most people figuratively "step aside" when he walks through. Not me. I'm not most people and neither are some of the paramedics that I'm proud to call colleagues.

As I look back on the differences of manhood, demeanor, leadership, and integrity between Colonel Dr. Shawn Michaels and Dr. Dipstick, I just shake my head in amazement. It's the difference between a Colonel and a Corporal. One could have been a Brigadier General and chose not to be. He didn't need a star on the collar of his shirt to prove to anyone what kind of man he is. The other craved a title that would bring him some sort of power as to perhaps recreate ambulance services in this county in his own image.

When I was a kid, we used to call other kids like him a punk, a sissy or a candy ass. As an adult you recognize it as the "Little-Big Man" syndrome. As paramedics who have to deal with this guy from time to time, we just refer to him as Corporal Candy Ass. It seems to fit perfectly.

Chapter 10
Corporal Candy Ass Becomes Major Pain

At the conclusion of that recorded phone call with the newly ordained Corporal Candy Ass, I knew I had gotten the best of him. He had clearly lost the intellectual argument in regard to the appropriate care given to this particular patient. However, the phone call itself did absolutely nothing for my disdain for him as a member of the human race let alone the medical profession.

For me it still didn't ease the pain and humiliation of him calling me a "danger to the community." The sting of seeing those words about me on paper is something I'll never forget. Consequently, he still remained a target for me, as much as I still remained a target for him. That would be more than fine with me.

My goal hadn't changed a bit. In a professional capacity, I would still be out to irritate him just as much as possible. As far as his insult to my personal integrity is concerned, that would be repaid in kind as well. Conversely, I could only imagine that he wasn't finished with me either. In his mind I'm sure he was just waiting for me to stick my neck out just far enough so he could give me a professional severing. I wouldn't have to wait a long time before there would be another incident to stir controversy and to stoke our incendiary relationship.

About thirty days after "the phone call," my most recent partner and long-time friend Gene and I responded to an emergency call to a private residence in Hartford. The request for help came to us at about 4 a.m. on a cold and snowy morning in February. The elderly woman complained of difficulty in breathing. When we arrived, the local fire department had responded to the lady's home with three or four men. They were there as medical first responders (MFR's) and as such had just placed oxygen on the woman.

The firemen had just finished recording a set of vital signs and had concluded their basic assessment when Gene and I walked through the door. They gave us a brief summation as to how upon their arrival the patient presented in general, her level of distress as to her ability to breathe adequately and finally a copy of her vital signs.

This particular fire department was comprised of a wonderful bunch of guys who like most other volunteer departments, have a great ethic and want to "give back" to their respective communities. So they are more than happy to do whatever they can for their fellow neighbors as well as to do anything they can for the responding ambulance team.

Although the training level in first-aid that most fire departments have attained doesn't approach the level of training a paramedic has acquired, we still very much appreciate the assistance they give to the patients prior to our arrival, on our behalf. Even if it is to just carry the ambulance cot and other equipment in and out of the house, the help they offer is great.

As Gene and I walked into the house, we saw an 83- year-old woman who looked to be generally healthy. She was able to walk without assistance from a cane or walker; however, she was standing and leaning with most of her body weight over a kitchen chair with an oxygen mask fitted snuggly in place. It was really easy to see and hear that she was really straining to breathe, and consequently could hardly talk. I immediately listened to her lung sounds with my stethoscope. I heard very mild wheezes and she was laboring against a whole lot of fluid in her lungs. To those who aren't aware of that significance, the short story is that when you have fluid in your lungs, it impairs the gas exchange between carbon dioxide and oxygen that must take place for you to breathe properly.

After putting our patient on oxygen the fire department personnel quickly rounded up her prescription medicines. It was obvious that she was currently being treated for congestive heart failure, (CHF). Eventually after about five minutes of breathing 100% oxygen, she felt considerably better. I really needed to ask her questions concerning her condition, but like I said, she couldn't adequately breathe, let alone talk. So I turned to her husband, who was just a couple of years younger than she was, and I asked him a few questions about her recent medical history. I asked him things like, when did her shortness of breath start? Was she still asleep when her breathing troubles started? Has her shortness of breath been that bad before today? Does she take all of her medicines as prescribed?

He was not very helpful at all. He was visibly upset with his wife for being sick! I thought to myself, what a butt head. There didn't seem to be any compassion toward his wife's entire struggle to breathe. After I listened to her lungs and heart tones, I took her blood pressure and my partner Gene recorded everything on our patient medical control forms.

I remember him asking me what her heart rate was. I told him that and her respiration rate as well. I told him that she was pale and slightly diaphoretic and I remember seeing him write all of this down. In the meantime, two of the MFR's had already retrieved our cot out of the ambulance and had brought it into the house.

By this time our patient felt much better and was questioning me as to whether she should still go to the hospital. I told her in no uncertain terms that although she felt better at the moment her underlying condition hadn't changed at all. I told her that if we took the oxygen off of her now that she would quickly find herself back in the same predicament as she was in when she summoned EMS for help.

At first she stated she wanted to "just wait awhile" and see how things turned out. When she said that I turned and looked at Gene, which was his cue to get involved in the debate. He gently touched her shoulder and said to her softly, "Ma'am, you really, really need to go now. It's clearly the right thing." That was it. That's all it took for her to go to the hospital, but not with us.

She absolutely insisted in going to the local Watervliet Community Hospital, with her husband, in their mini-van. We urged her in vain to go with us in the ambulance. She wouldn't hear of it. I don't know whether it was the money issue, the idea of being in an ambulance, or what. We told her that she needed to be closely monitored with our Life Pack cardiac monitor, oxygen would have to be continued, an IV would have to be started and medicine would have to be administered as to improve her condition in a meaningful way.

Gene even told her that we had to drive right by the hospital on our way back to our ambulance station, so it would be no trouble for us at all. I chimed in and told her that I was extremely uncomfortable with her going to the hospital on her own. That's when she said that her husband could take her.

We continued to try to reason with her to the point that it was clearly starting to upset her.

When that started, I quit talking and said, "Okay, how about if we at least help you to your van?"

She nodded her head in agreement. I motioned to the firemen that they could return the cot to the ambulance and the lady and I walked out of her house with the portable oxygen bottle in hand. At this point in time, I didn't want to waste any more time with not getting her to the local emergency room with a protracted debate. Her husband had brushed the snow off the mini-van, that he had idling in an attempt to warm it.

As we walked slowly to the van, I just spoke softly to her and told her that we were here to help in any way that we can and that we would be following her to the hospital with the ambulance, just in case things took a turn for the worse with her. She acknowledged by just shaking her head, but didn't say a word. As we approached the van, I took the oxygen off of her.

She was clearly short of breath again. That was no surprise at all. It was probably about forty to fifty feet in ankle deep snow to where her chosen ride was awaiting her.

After I got her seated and spun her legs into the van I said, "Listen to me, it's not too late. I can still take you with me if you wish."

By this time she was again panting but still managed to simply say, "Thank you, no."

As Gene and I climbed into the ambulance, I told him how rapidly her condition had deteriorated.

Being slightly alarmed at my statement he immediately said to me, "I know, but what are you supposed to do? For God's sake, we can't kidnap her!"

Gene was of course correct. We cannot and do not just throw people on our cot who can legitimately speak for themselves. The bottom line is no matter what your condition is, you don't have to seek medical attention if you don't want it.

This incident reminded me of a call I had been on in the past.

I hadn't been in EMS for more than a year, when I had responded to the home of a guy who was a widower. He was living alone in a small house in the city of Bridgman. I don't recall who called us, but when we arrived there was a most peculiar odor emanating from the old man's house. After a lengthy career in the business of EMS, I now know that odor as gangrene.

As my partner and I walked into the house along with a city cop, I saw a man by the name of Mr. Gower sitting in his kitchen. He was on a chair, with his feet resting on an open electric oven door that he was using for heat. Both of his feet were wrapped in what looked like dirty, and body-fluid soaked gauze bandages.

Through his haphazardly wrapped feet, you could see that although he was a Caucasian man, his feet were solid black, right up to his ankles. Even being relatively new to the business, it didn't take a trained eye to see that he was going to die soon or he was going to lose his feet, or both.

We looked at his general living condition and talked with him for a while and said to him that we needed to take him to the hospital. He then says to the three of us, that he doesn't want to go.

I said to him, "Mr. Gower, you have to go. Look at your feet!"

The cranky old guy looks up at me and says, "I don't wanna go and get out of my house!"

I turned to the small town city cop who was standing right next to me and I said to him, "Can you make him go? He really needs to be in the hospital."

Without directly answering me, he leans down to Mr. Gower and says, "Mr. Gower, sir, you really need to go to the hospital."

Mr. Gower gives the cop the same answer as he gave me: "No I don't and you get out of my house, too."

Well we just couldn't just leave him there so the cop calls the chief of police over to the house and gives him the story and the chief has no better luck convincing Mr. Gower and his two rotting feet to go to the hospital. So the chief makes a call to the prosecuting attorney for our county and gave him the same story. The prosecuting attorney (who later became the U.S. Attorney for the Western District of Michigan) said that if Mr. Gower is of sound mind, he doesn't have to do anything he doesn't want to do. Period. End of story.

Through the years, I've never forgotten that. I don't recall now what ever happened to that old geezer, but I'm fairly certain he didn't last too long after my short visit with him. Being of sound mind just means you know who you are, where you are and what time of the day, week or year that it is. It doesn't mean that you have to agree with the vast majority of people who think differently than you do in general or your medical decisions, and your well being in particular.

So, even though Gene and I both knew that this nice, elderly and very sick lady really would have greatly benefited from our expert services, in the end, "no" still meant "no." As promised, we did follow her and her husband right up to the point as to where they turned onto the hospital driveway and we continued on to our station, satisfied in the fact that we did everything that we could reasonably do for the lady.

As he and I are retiring to our respective bedrooms, the staff at the Watervliet hospital was having a full tilt conniption fit. After all, this lady presented to them as having profound shortness of breath, secondary to severe congestive heart failure. They of course found out there was an ambulance on the scene and the ambulance personnel didn't take her to the hospital.

Well after everything was said and done, the lady was admitted to their Intensive Care Unit at the local community hospital. Although it sounds serious, it's not really all that bad because anybody with more than the sniffles ends up being transferred out of that small community hospital to be taken to Borgess Hospital in Kalamazoo.

When I found out later that she hadn't been transferred, I wasn't that impressed. As the story goes, Cpl. Candy Ass gets on the case and wants to know why she didn't come in by ambulance and who was on duty and who didn't bring her in. When the good doctor found out it was me on this call, he had his mission. So he gets on the phone to our new Project Medical Director (PMD), Doctor Royale and says that he wants to know what happened and why I didn't take her to the hospital and where was the paper work with this whole matter?

As fate would have it, when Gene got up to go home, he forgot to get the dispatch times on this call. I didn't think anything of it because Gene said earlier in the morning, when we got back to our station that he was going to handle it. Since Gene was doing the specific paperwork that is required for those patient's that we see and or treat but don't transport I didn't think anything more about it.

After all, the woman made it to the hospital and I felt confident in saying that we did our level best in attempting to convince her to go with us. She finally got the care she desperately needed and everything is good. Right? Wrong!

When we both got up that fateful morning to leave the station little did we know that would be the last call of Gene's career in EMS. During the last couple of years or so, Gene had filed a lawsuit against Medic 1 Ambulance in district court as well as one in Federal court.

He and his lawyer settled both lawsuits and one of the stipulations for settlement was that he not be employed at Medic 1 Ambulance from that day, forward. So, as luck would have it, that day was Gene's last day and he was unconcerned about anything to do with Medic 1. He had his day in court, got his settlement and was gone.

One day a couple of weeks after this latest incident, Dr. Royale sees me doing paperwork in the paramedic room just outside the entry to the emergency room. So he approaches me and we start to talk yet again about this same call. As we are talking, Doctor Royale says that he called Gene and Gene said in no uncertain terms that he no longer worked for Medic 1 and to go take a flying leap.

So he comes back to me and says, "Nimtz isn't going to help us in Dr. Dipstick's concerns, so it's up to you."

"Hold on there doc, just because you can't find the paperwork that I saw Gene filling out during that call, doesn't mean I'm now somehow responsible for it just because he no longer is employed here."

"Yes it does."

"No it doesn't! I'm not, nor was I ever his supervisor, so, no it doesn't!"

"Well, you're the only one left."

"Well, I can't help you with that so I don't know what you want me to say. I don't have the paperwork. Nor did I ever have it. I saw Gene writing it out, but that was the closest that I came to having it. If I were to guess, I would think that Gene took it home with him by accident with all of the newspapers he looks through everyday and probably threw it out in the trash."

Dr. Royale hesitates for a moment and then says to me, "Well Gene has made it abundantly clear that he will not help in this matter. So now you're stuck with it."

At this time I can feel myself starting to boil. "Listen here doc, like I said, I never had it, I don't know where it is and since I was not Gene's supervisor, I absolutely refuse to be responsible for him."

Dr. Royale shrugs his shoulders and says, "Well Dr. Dipstick wants to have a meeting about it."

"Well of course he does. He's an asshole and he's got you running around in circles for him!"

"Well Jim, we just have to make sure everything is done properly, that's all."

"Well that's bullshit and we all know it, so spare me. In fact, tell Cpl. Candy Ass to take his best shot."

I hesitated for a moment wondering and waiting to see what Dr. Royale was going to say about me telling him Cpl. Candy Ass has him running around in circles.

He didn't say anything. So I continued, "You know doc, with all of the problems you could be fixing in EMS in this county with a couple of the ambulance services that you know are violating real and meaningful rules and regulations, it's a shame that you focus on a meeting about a call that I ran on, that had no consequences to it at all. You know it and so do I. Furthermore, you know that your buddy from Watervliet knows it too. This is just another attempt to twist me. Like I said, you can tell that little sissy bastard for me, to take his best shot."

Dr. Royale just gives me that "oh well" look, and starts to walk away.

I then quickly add, "Hey doc, tell that little punk that I carry my paramedic license in my wallet. If he can get to it, he can have it!"

Dr. Royale just smiles and says as he's walking away, "I don't think he'll want to do that."

So while I'm finishing up with the paperwork that I'm filling out on about the millionth patient I've seen over the years, I'm thinking to myself, "I sure hope I'm irritating the hell out of that asshole because he sure is irritating the hell out of me."

As divine providence would have it, there would be yet another incident involving me that would send Dr. Dipstick into an absolute frenzy.

***

The local racetrack in Hartford was just starting their Friday night racing season. Practice racing and testing and tuning dates had been rained out in the previous weeks, so this is everybody's first racing of the season. The racetrack is a 5/8 of a mile long oval clay track and they race everything from factory stocks right up to the Outlaw sprint cars.

At that time the two brothers and their families who owned and operated the dirt track did a fine job and they usually put on several hours of great entertainment for just a few dollars. They consistently contracted with Medic 1 to have an ambulance at the track whenever there was racing. Their racing season usually started in early to mid April. It was every Friday night (weather permitting) until Labor Day.

On that particular first Friday night of racing, local history was going to be made as Dave Tober and his daughter Allison were set to be the first father/daughter racers to take their place along side many other racers that night. The Tobers were a multigenerational family of racers that started with Dave's father. Dave was set to race the silver #14 and Allison, the purple and white #14 factory stock cars.

For several years my partner, John Hubbard and I almost exclusively did the weekly standby at the track and were looking forward to the new season. I know that the two brothers who contracted with Medic 1 to have an ambulance at their track, regularly told John and me that they really appreciated having the same two guys each and every week.

The local fire crew at the track appreciated it as well. It's just that most people are more comfortable with familiarity as opposed to having different people there each Friday night. Everything was going as planned and John and I are watching these guys going around in counterclockwise circles and having just a good 'ole time.

They were getting into the main feature races for all of the different classes of racing and the factory stocks were running around the track as best as they could hoping a wheel didn't fall off. That's when John pointed out that the driver of car #14 appeared to have been stopping. We just watched him slow down to a stop as he just kind of "clunked" into the inside guard rail of the track. I remember thinking to myself that was really odd. Did he just run out of gas? Did his drive shaft come off? Did his steering wheel or something else break or what?

The flagman flipped on the yellow caution light and set out the yellow flag. At that moment the fire department personnel that run the track as the safety crew, rode their specially equipped pick-up truck out onto the track to attempt to quickly remedy any problem that a driver or car may be experiencing.

When they got next to the disabled car they checked on the status of the driver before they do anything else. Almost immediately, three out of the five guys on the safety crew started to do what looked like jumping jacks, in an attempt to get us out onto the track. John fired up the ambulance and we got out to where the car had appeared to have just simply stalled.

We jumped out of the ambulance and discovered that the driver, Dave Tober had in fact lost consciousness. We quickly found that he was having deep snoring respirations and was cyanotic (blue) in color. I'm thinking right away that this guy has had a brain injury, and I'm certain it wasn't from racing. It was clear to us that no other car touched him. John called dispatch and our dispatcher called for the Watervliet stationed Medic 1 ambulance to come to the racetrack.

The protocol is that John and I take care of the problem and then the local service ambulance does the transporting. As he is doing that the firefighters and I wondered how we were going to get this big guy out of his car. The doors are welded shut and he has a roll cage around him.

To top it all off, he's got one of those specially designed seats that looked to be wrapped around him on three sides. Dave was a big, husky guy, who according to his family was six-foot three inches tall and weighed maybe 280 pounds. He was wearing a heavy fire retardant, one piece racing suit and a big full-faced helmet.

We simply couldn't pull Dave out through one of his windows and he appears to be essentially dying right in front of us. The only chance to save his life would be to cut the sheet metal off of the top of his car and pull him up and straight through the roof of his car. That's what we did.

I wasn't concerned at all with his neck—or as we say, cervical spine—because John and I knew that what happened to this guy was not traumatic. We were absolutely certain it was organic. After the sheet metal was removed from the roof of the car, we still put the KED board (a type of "wrap-around backboard) in place and fastened it to him just so all of the rescuers at this man's side would have something to grab onto to lift him out of his car.

Before we removed him and while the firemen were busy cutting the top of the car off, I was getting his gloves, helmet and hood off of him to better assess him. When I finally was able to assess him, he was in worse shape than I had initially thought.

His pupils were unequal, and he had no reaction to pain at all. He was still cyanotic but not as bad as he had been because John had secured an oxygen mask onto his face, by lifting the visor to his helmet right after we had gotten to his car. For whatever reason, he was profoundly unconscious and I intuitively knew that he had suffered some sort of insult to his brain.

By the time we had removed Dave from his car the ambulance had arrived and we got the driver lying supine on our ambulance cot. We started out by cutting his racing clothes off of him and initiated our full assessment of his level of consciousness. John was reassessing his airway and adjusting the amount of oxygen he was giving him. Bob, another paramedic, was getting our patient onto our cardiac monitor and I was looking to start an IV. Just as I'm ready to stick him with the needle, I noticed that our patient started to exhibit a decerebrate posture.

A decerebrate posture means that his arms and legs are fully extended, and he is trying to twist them inward. It looks like the backsides of our patient's hands would be touching the lateral sides of his thighs. The feet would be twisting in the same fashion. What it essentially means for the stricken patient is that he has suffered a catastrophic brain injury. It is usually a severe enough insult to the brain, which in all likelihood will turn out to be fatal for most people.

When he started that type of posturing, I immediately said, "Guys, he's decerebrating! We've got to go right now!" I looked at Bob and his partner Jerry and I said, "He's got to go to Lakeland right now!"

By the look on Bob's face, he didn't want anything to do with this guy. I can't say that I blamed him. Here, he and his EMT partner came to do a simple transport to the local facility, which is only four or five miles away. Instead, they find themselves in the middle of an extremely critical situation, where the closest appropriate hospital is roughly twenty miles from the racetrack. I can't honestly say that I would have been too keen on the idea if I had been in their shoes.

I know that Jerry is a basic EMT and therefore the designated driver, so I made the decision and said to the guys, "I'll tell you what. Bob, you stay here at the racetrack with John. Jerry, you get in that front seat and when you get us to I-94, you go as fast as this bucket will go and get us to Lakeland!"

So, that's what happened. The track is about two miles from the highway and it's about eighteen minutes to that particular hospital from there.

Although the incident was tragic in nature, there were really two great things that happened as far as I was personally concerned. First and foremost, I bypassed the Watervliet hospital that was only a few miles from the racetrack and elected to travel more than twenty miles to Lakeland Hospital. I knew there was a neurosurgeon on duty at the time at Lakeland, whereas Watervliet had no such thing.

It had been my experience over the years and utmost belief that if you take someone to a facility where they cannot give definitive care in a reasonable amount of time, you might as well leave them laying on the "kitchen floor," or in this case, in the race car. The only thing that the Watervliet hospital would have done other than ring the cash register, would be to call for our patient to be taken by helicopter to Borgess or Bronson hospitals in Kalamazoo. By all of our patient's signs and symptoms what our patient needed was a neurosurgeon that very minute.

On the way to the highway, Jerry asked me if I was going to call Watervliet and get their permission to bypass their treatment center and go directly to Lakeland Hospital. I told Jerry that I wouldn't have time to get their "permission." I told him that my time would be better spent saving this man's life. Without a doubt I knew that it was first and foremost, exactly the right thing to do.

I knew Dr. Dipstick would really have his nose out of joint over this emergency. I knew he would be just furious. (Did I mention that would be perfectly fine with me?) During this time, I was as busy as I could possibly be checking and rechecking vital signs, lung sounds, and neurological status.

Through it all, I came to the conclusion that his condition had somewhat stabilized. I thought about intubating him, but he seemed to be breathing fine with the non re-breather oxygen mask in place. In retrospect I probably should have intubated him as a protective measure against a potentially compromised airway.

His EKG looked normal and I had started the IV that I had put off for the moment back at the racetrack. Through continuous assessment, I was confident that he would make it alive to the hospital. I was equally sure that his long-term survival would be slim, at best.

Now, before I go any further, I have to tell you that bypassing the local hospital, even though it could be of little help to our patient, is not what most people in EMS would have done. Why? It is simply less trouble for the ambulance team. They would get rid of a very critical patient and now it's somebody else's problem. My problem with that train of thought is that it doesn't do a whole lot of good for the patient! I can honestly state that I have always in times of great need, like this call, been willing to extend myself with decision making and treatment that is on the edge. I guess it's just the way that I'm wired.

As the ambulance is rocketing down I-94, I contacted Lakeland Hospital in St. Joseph twice. The first time was to let them know of the patient we were bringing to them and of his emergent condition. The second time was to reiterate the seriousness of this patient's condition and that they had better be ready and that they could expect us in three to four minutes.

When we roared into the ambulance garage, I saw Dr. Royale come running out into the garage with a couple of nurses, which is really unusual.

I threw open the back doors of the ambulance and immediately said to him, "Doc, he's posturing and his pupils were unequal earlier."

As Dr. Royale quickly is assessing my patient, I can almost see him thinking. Of course, he knows full well what the fallout of this is going to be with Cpl. Candy Ass throwing another snit.

"Jim, I don't have a problem with what you did (by bringing the patient here instead of Watervliet), but why did it have to be you?" Dr. Royale said.

Well, I was exactly right.

"Oh doc, you're missing the point," I said. "I wanted it to be me. I'm glad it was me. I want to get under this guy's skin whenever I can. I want to irritate him however and whenever I possibly can!"

The fact is, that I wanted to trivialize him as much as possible while still delivering top-notch, pre-hospital, emergency medical care. I still wanted to disrespect him however, and whenever I could. I despised his pseudo-authority and his little "fiefdom" in Watervliet. On my part, with my decision to take my very critically ill patient to a hospital fifteen miles further away from the closest facility, some may call it foolhardy. I choose to call it going to the closest hospital that would be able to address his medical needs. The distant second, but very tangible and personally great thing about this call was the certainty of Cpl. Candy Ass losing his mind over this particular medical emergency and knowing that I, his arch nemesis, made the call without consulting him or his minions in his emergency room.

***

In the five to six weeks in between the two calls that I had just mentioned, a committee meeting was set to review the call about the lady who Gene and I had unsuccessfully urged to go to the hospital with us. It seems as though Dr. Royale had bowed to the wishes of Cpl. Candy Ass. As it turned out John, my partner at the track was a member on that particular committee representing the interests of Medic 1.

I told the committee members what had happened and explained to them line and verse what had transpired. I told them what we saw, and how Gene and I implored her to go with us to the hospital. I also told them that we had followed her to the hospital just in case we were needed at any time.

None of it sat well with Dr. Dipstick, and he told me as much. I, in kind, told him that I didn't give a damn what he thought or why. The problem was the missing paperwork. That was long gone and nothing was going to bring it back. Even after I told them how I saw Gene writing out the facts as I listed them to him, they still thought that I was responsible just because they couldn't get to Gene. It was the most ridiculous thing I had ever heard.

Subsequent to hearing everything I had to say, they kicked me out of the meeting so they could talk about me. I waited for more than ninety minutes just to hear them come to the conclusion that they couldn't find me at fault. Immediately following the closed conversation, I learned from one of the participants that during their sequestered debate, Cpl. Candy Ass told the committee that I should be disciplined because I showed a "pattern of bad judgment", referring to the subsequent issues.

Knowing full well that this meeting was to discuss this call with the elderly lady and only this call, I was just livid that he, being the smarmy bastard that he is, would try to bring in other unrelated issues.

He had thrown the gauntlet down and I was now prepared to pick it up and beat him with it! I came back into the same meeting room in which I had just left five minutes earlier to find Dr. Royale and Corporal Candy Ass standing and having a conversation. Nobody else was in the room.

As I approached the two of them, I turned to my arch nemesis and said to him, "I heard you brought up the ambulance call from last September, why? Tell me why, you bastard!"

Dr. Royale immediately says to me, "Calm down Jim!"

I retort, "I can't calm down! This cocksucker right here hasn't got the balls to bring this bullshit up while I'm in front of him. This motherfucker has to do it behind my back!"

Now as I approached him I start to cuss and scream at the top of my lungs until I am literally six inches from his face. Now we are face-to-face and I am verbally lighting him up. As much as it pains me to say, he only took one step backwards as I approached him. I'm not at all proud of the fact that I said the things that I did. Up until that day, I had never said those words to any person, ever.

I know now that I was really in a fit of rage and just barely under enough self-control not to strike him physically. I have never in all my years wanted to kick the hell out of anyone as bad as I did that day. I knew that if he had so much as nudged me, he would have gotten the beating of a lifetime. He knew that as well.

For him it would have been a hospital bed, and for me the county jail. Understand that my work is my life's passion and this man was trying to defame me to my peers and colleagues because my decisions bruised his ego.

As badly as I wanted to hurt him physically, it wouldn't have been worth the trouble. After all, he didn't violate one of my children or even kick one of my beloved long-haired dachshunds. He just tried to get me fired from my job. So after about a thirty-second tongue lashing, in which he didn't say a single word, I turned from him and stormed out of the meeting room slamming the door as hard as I could. As I was leaving the hospital, I remember just shaking for about five minutes. After that, I was maybe just as calm and as relaxed as I have ever been. The whole episode was cathartic in nature.

As the days and weeks rolled by, there were subtle signs that he was still after me. One of my trusted friends and fellow paramedic, Bob White, wrote me a memo that said he had a most peculiar discussion with Dr. Dipstick right after he and his partner had transported a patient to the Watervliet hospital's emergency room. The doctor had questioned my friend on whether or not I was a "good" paramedic.

He asked whether I had any trouble with any other medical people, colleagues, etc. Bob told me in his memo that he thought the time he spent talking with him was just plain weird to the point of being uncomfortable. The bottom-line, my colleague told me to watch my back.

As this feud continued to escalate, Dr. Royale said that it all was going before the county medical control board and I had better bring a lawyer with me. I told him that there would be no problem with that and that I was looking forward to arguing my case in front of his and Corporal Candy Ass's colleagues.

During this whole time, I had piqued the interest of a few doctors in the emergency room at Lakeland Hospital, our main hospital. They knew about the conflict and how it was escalating. They understood what I was doing as far as being a continual irritant to the chronic whiner from Watervliet.

One of my doctor supporters was a guy by the name of Dr. Bob Stephen. He knew all about the unending hostility and told me, "I had better be really careful." He also told me that I had his support and that if I needed him for whatever reason, I was to call him.

The former PMD, Dr. Kraff just couldn't believe how I was being treated and why. He likewise told me that I could count on his support as well. In the meantime, I found out that my cousin's wife was a labor attorney and that she worked for some big outfit from Kalamazoo. I knew that Stacy was an attorney, but I didn't know that she would be the one to help me out. After my wife and I made a dinner appointment with Stacy, and told her of the antics of this putz, she said she would be glad to represent me and put this little Napoleon wanna-be in his place.

Stacey told me that the best thing I could do was to call Dr. Dipstick and attempt to resolve the issue between us if it were possible. Although I know it was sound, it really galled me to acquiesce to her counsel. Although I didn't overtly shun my lawyer's advice and as I talked with him on the phone, I didn't make a good faith effort to resolve the issue. That would have meant that I would have had to say that I'm sorry.

I've never had a problem in the past, nor do I have a problem now saying, "I'm sorry" or issuing an apology if I'm in error. But I didn't' make a mistake or misstep about any of it. It was Corporal Candy Ass who was in error from the very beginning. There is no doubt whatsoever that he made errors of assumption, of patient care, of EMS protocols and lastly and perhaps most importantly, of self-determination.

After that incident on the phone and during my subsequent events, I had talked to Stacy about six to eight times and kept her apprised of my situation. Finally, Dr. Royale saw me at the hospital during an early morning call and informed me that a meeting date was now set. I told him I was glad to hear it and that my lawyer and I would certainly be in attendance. I remember being really confident, but still a little nervous. After all, my professional life as a paramedic was now on the line.

As the day approached, my friend Gene contacted me and said that he had heard through the grapevine that there was a big meeting set. I told him he was correct and that he ought to help me out. He quickly agreed and before I knew it, Stacy had received a letter in the mail from Gene. He explained to her the whole call in reference to the elderly lady with the difficulty breathing who wouldn't go to the hospital with us.

What was really nice was that Gene also wrote a cover letter that explained from his point of view, my knowledge, expertise, and experience in handling medical emergencies. And also about the feud that was well known by most everybody who works in the local emergency room, as well as EMS people in our area. He told Stacy that the only reason any of this was going as far as it had, was because I didn't give the doctor the respect and deference that he thought he was due. He knew, as we all knew, that this whole fiasco was not event-driven but anger and ego-driven.

As Gene was writing his letter, I was lining up Dr. Kraff and Dr. Stephen.

I remember Dr. Stephen saying to me in an unbelieving tone, "All of this is really going to go to the medical control authority board? That's really idiotic."

He couldn't believe that Dr. Dipstick was still pushing this issue. Anyway, both of them told me that they would absolutely be there.

Just before the mid morning meeting got underway, Gene, Stacy and my doctor supporters and I met to discuss the pertinent aspects of the meeting and who was going to say what to whom and so forth. The common thread to each of our thinking was that this whole thing was trivial in nature and lacked good sense or intelligence in the extreme.

Up to this point, I had never seen doctors express even minor disagreements with each other—at least not outwardly, let alone publicly. They seemed to always support and "cover" each other. But here we are with at least two highly respected doctors who are willing and almost eager to come to the cause of a seasoned and highly experienced paramedic.

As we were talking outside the meeting room, one of the committee members opened the door and said, "The committee is waiting for you."

As we walked into the room, Gene was first, then me, Stacy and lastly, the doctors. Dr. Royale was the chairman of the committee and he started off by thanking everybody for taking the time to attend this important meeting and that I wouldn't be the only item on the agenda. He got started by stating the facts, as he understood them and the concerns of Dr. Dipstick's. Anyone could tell that Dr. Royale was attempting to walk a tightrope and was struggling just a bit.

Almost immediately he started to ask me questions about his concerns of my judgment and possible fine points of protocol violations. Stacy immediately interrupted him and asked whether or not other paramedics undergo such scrutiny. She reminds him of other possible protocol violations that haven't been addressed and standard operating procedures (SOP) that are technically not within our stated protocols. Week's prior, I gave Stacy all of the manuals regarding Medic 1 operations, employees and pre-hospital medicine. In all, it probably was more than a thousand pages that she poured through in preparation for this meeting.

When Stacy and Dr. Royale were done bantering it was Cpl. Candy Ass's turn. Instead of him saying anything directly to me, he had one of his physician assistants (lackeys) do his talking for him. It was just as well, because I would have been incredibly hostile toward him and most likely all the key players at the meeting knew it as well.

The assistant asked me why I did this or why I didn't do that as far as the race car driver was concerned. That was of course after they asked Gene about the call regarding the elderly lady whose paperwork had turned up missing. Gene sat there and told the committee point blank and as a whole that he filled out the required paperwork. He forgot to get the dispatch times to be recorded and subsequently was to blame for losing the paperwork. Furthermore, he stated that he thought that it was utterly ridiculous that I should be or would be held responsible for his mishap.

Finally, he told the committee that he did not intend to address the subject again and as far as he was concerned, it was a dead issue. The assistant then started out by laser focusing on the course of treatment and the unilateral decision I had made about bi-passing the closest hospital. He did so by suggesting that I had taken other patients with head injuries to the Watervliet hospital as well as other seriously injured or ill patients.

I said that I had never, nor would I ever entertain the thought of taking someone to Watervliet Community Hospital who was in dire need of a neurosurgeon. I told everyone in attendance, what they—in their hearts and minds—already knew. It makes no sense in the realm of morbidity, as well as mortality that a patient should be taken to a hospital where definitive care cannot be achieved. The only thing that would have a snowball's chance in hell in helping someone in that condition was surgical intervention. A small community hospital just doesn't even have a neurosurgeon on call, let alone one on staff. That fact isn't going to change, even with Attila the Hun running the emergency room.

Dr. Stephen piped up and said, "I have sat here for the last twenty minutes and I have yet to hear anything that would suggest that this meeting was needed. I also think that what Jim did on behalf of this particular patient was exactly the right thing to do."

"You can say for sure that Jim knew for sure that there was a neurosurgeon on call that night?" Cpl. Candy Ass said, now speaking for himself.

"Yes, I can," he said assuredly. "What doctors are on call and their specialty are posted for all to see. In fact the neurosurgeon is in the hospital right now. If I need him, he's only two minutes away."

As I listened to Dr. Stephen dress down the sissy from Watervliet, I thought to myself, I have never, in my life, ever heard doctors trading verbal punches like this! If that weren't enough, Dr. Kraff must have heard enough because he started in immediately with his thoughts on the whole issue and how idiotic it all was.

"I think we all know in our heart of hearts that none of us would be here in this meeting today if it weren't Jim Stine being the one in question," Dr. Kraff said definitively. "There are simply no grounds for any of this. C'mon, we all know this is silly."

"I resent that!" Cpl. Candy Ass blurted.

"You know he's right you son-of-a-bitch!" I said sticking up for the doctor.

At that moment, Stacy grabbed my arm and nearly shook it off of the table. "Shhhhhh, don't you say anything unless I tell you to!" she commanded.

Dr. Royale quickly got the meeting back in order. Stacy reiterated how all of this complaining from one person has to be from a personal vendetta and nothing more. After that and what Gene said about the first call regarding the little old lady who wouldn't go to the hospital by ambulance, and how Drs. Stephen and Kraff just slammed the door on the face of Cpl. Candy Ass, it was pretty much a done deal. And that the whole issue of me being suspended, fired or my license revoked was now dead in the water.

At that time, I think Dr. Royale knew it as well. This whole sorry episode was putting the egg on too many faces so Dr. Royale called for a committee decision. My team was politely asked to leave the room while they contemplated what had been said, and render a decision. As the five of us walked out of the meeting room we collectively decided to get something to drink in the little café just down the hallway from the meeting room and discuss what had just transpired.

I immediately took time to thank the doctors for standing up for me. I told them both, they really unhinged Cpl. Candy Ass's case against me and put it into proper context for all to see. Stacy was magnificent in her defensive posture as she argued each and every point as to put me in the most favorable light as I was being dragged through the mud.

For me, the thing that encapsulates this whole sorry episode was what Dr. Kraff said while we were sitting there in the café waiting for the medical control committee's decision.

He said, "If it doesn't end here, today, I think there should be money involved."

If I ever thought that I might live to be a thousand, I never thought that I would ever hear one doctor advocating bringing a lawsuit against another doctor. It was an amazing statement.

We only waited for maybe twenty-five minutes and then we were asked to rejoin the meeting. As expected they found no cause for discipline for any of the complaints brought by Corporal Candy Ass or his minions.

***

Not long after the mother of all meetings had concluded, I was again working at our Watervliet station during one of my scheduled twenty-four hour shifts with a guy by the name of Mike Kushman. At approximately 1:40 a.m., we received a call for an elderly lady with chest discomfort. Fortunately for her she only lived about a mile from our station.

When we arrived, we found this very nice and very plump 73-year-old lady complaining of chest pain that started about two days ago. She said that it went away but had returned the previous afternoon and within the last five to six hours was getting progressively more uncomfortable.

I immediately sent Mike out to get the ambulance cot and told him to bring the oxygen in to her. While he was busy doing that, I was doing a cardiac related assessment, obtaining her medical history, and was busy looking over what type of prescription drugs she was taking on a daily basis and so forth. It only took about three minutes for Mike to get back into the house, at which time he quickly put a nasal cannula on our patient and gave her 4L/min. of oxygen.

He said that due to the narrowness of the entry point of her house that he wouldn't be able to get the cot through the door. At this time I had ascertained that the lady we were treating in all likelihood was in the process of suffering a heart attack. After recording her vital signs and listening to her lung sounds and placing her on oxygen, we helped her to our ambulance cot.

Once we got her secured to our cot, I gave her a dose of sublingual nitroglycerin. We then hustled her out to the ambulance where Mike hooked her up to our cardiac monitor and reassessed her oxygen needs to make her as comfortable as possible. I quickly gave her four 81mg. tablets of aspirin and told her to just chew them up and to let them dissolve in her mouth.

I started an IV and then told Mike that I thought that we were ready for our three-minute ride to the Watervliet hospital. During the trip, I questioned her about her chest pain. She said that although she felt "better," the pain was still there. Since her blood pressure was still well within normal limits, I gave her another spritz of nitroglycerin under her tongue.

Mike had just pulled the ambulance up to the emergency room entrance and we quickly got her through the door and onto a hospital bed in one of the rooms in the emergency department. She hadn't been on the hospital gurney for more than thirty seconds, and while I was giving a medical report to one of the three attending nurses, our lady suddenly turns reddish-purple. She began making a sound like she's letting air out of a tire. It looked like every single muscle in her body was in spasm.

"She's going into cardiac arrest! She's going into cardiac arrest!" I yelled to the nurses.

"Jim, does she have a history of seizures?" one asked.

I immediately think to myself, Don't you as an emergency room registered nurse even recognize the arrival of clinical death when you see it? Instead I just yelled, "No! I'm telling you, she's going into arrest!"

One of the other attending nurses yells out to the doctor on duty, "Dr. Jones, Dr. Jones!"

Suddenly, Dr. "Jones" comes running through the door, quickly looks at the patient and says to me, "Jim, does she have a history of seizures?"

Although all of this happened in just the span of approximately forty seconds, I found myself just about ready to bleed out of my eyeballs! I immediately grabbed her wrist and shook it toward our unknowing hospital medical staff and said, "Doc, I'm telling you I don't have anything here! She's in arrest!"

"Well let's get her on the monitor," the doctor ordered.

I thought to myself in disdain, "What a novel thought. Yeah, let's put the cardiac monitor on her."

Once the monitor was turned on it showed that our lady was, indeed, in cardiac arrest.

"We better shock that!" the doctor ordered.

Again, I think, "What a novel idea."

In the meantime, there was a somewhat older nurse between the defibrillator and me. She looked at the array of buttons on the machine and just started pushing all of them in an attempt to charge up the defibrillator so she could shock the poor woman's heart.

After watching her push just about every button twice, I said to her, "Watch out. Let me do this."

I gently nudged her out of the way, quickly looked over the machine and noticed the only thing that the nurse didn't touch... the dial that measures out the intensity of the shock to be delivered to the patient's heart. It was a set at zero. Obviously, nothing will charge if the energy to be delivered is zero.

So I ratcheted up the dial to 300 watts and then hit the charge button. I seized the defibrillator paddles, demanding defib gel. The same nurse who couldn't operate the machine, grabbed the large tube of gel, fumbled it and the doctor caught it in mid air. He opened the tube and quickly squirted about a teaspoon out onto one of the paddles that I was holding. I then rubbed them together and told everybody to clear away from the patient. I made sure everyone was out of the way and then zapped the patient right back into a regular sinus rhythm, which is a regular EKG heart pattern.

Dr. Jones then says, "Let's get her intubated."

Since I love to intubate patients, I snapped at the chance, saying, "I'll do that right now for you, doc."

He quickly added, "Well I want to knock her down with some morphine and versed."

He turned to the younger of the three nurses and asked for 15mg. of morphine and 5mg. of versed. As she headed to the locked cabinet to get the medicine, I had intubated the patient to protect her airway. One minute or so later she started to regain consciousness and then started to "buck" the tube. ("Bucking the tube," means that it appears the patient is choking on it and tries to cough or expel the tube).

As all of this is happening, the young nurse yelled out, "I can't find the versed!"

I immediately yelled out, "Look under Midazolam!"

"Oh, here it is!" she yells back.

Now, as the patient is fighting the tube that I just put into her trachea, another nurse starts arguing with me that I have the tube in her esophagus (which would be in the wrong place, because that, of course, leads to the stomach and not the lungs). I told the nurse that was trying to tell me how to manage this patient's airway that this type of reaction to endo-tracheal tube placement is normal, and the only thing we had to do for her would be to breath for her by using our "Ambu-bag."

It's been my vast experience over the years that if you "bag" someone who is in a semi-conscious state, that after the fourth or fifth time you breathe for the patient, they calm down and everything is fine. Of course, the nurse didn't believe that. She wants me to pull the tube out and re-intubate the patient. Of course that wasn't going to happen.

So instead, I just grabbed the bag out of the nurse's hand and proceeded to squeeze it four to five times, ventilating her over a twenty-second period. The patient was still uncomfortable and would stay that way until the other nurse figured out how to give the right medication that the doctor ordered. For me, the patient was now manageable, with a minimal amount of trouble. The nurses finally got the morphine and versed into the patient, and she was now adequately sedated so her medical care would be easier to administer.

Let us look at this particular patient's care and see what had transpired:
1. The paramedic recognized a witnessed cardiac arrest when one doctor and three nurses erroneously thought she was suffering a grand mal seizure.

2. The paramedic defibrillated the patient while the older nurse tried to and couldn't figure out how to operate the machine in a timely fashion.

3. The paramedic told the younger nurse the generic name for versed (which is how they are listed most of the time in the hospital setting) because she didn't know.

4. The paramedic intubated her and managed her airway so the patient would be assured of being able to breathe adequately. Mike then took over the care and mainte-nance of her oxygen administration and ventilation to control her rate of breathing.

To think that we had to come to the rescue of a lady having a heart attack is, and should be no big deal. It's what we are precisely trained to do. The idea of having to do this in the middle of an emergency room with a doctor and at least three nurses present is inexcusable and frightening, not to mention almost unbelievable.

As Mike and I relinquished care for our patient to the hospital staff, I was happy that we were able to do the good things that we did. At the same time, I was angry and incredulous to the fact that, I'm the guy who's supposed to be "a danger to the community". The indisputable fact is that Mike and I outright saved this woman's life right in the middle of Corporal Candy Ass's own emergency room.

Mike and I finally left the emergency room shortly after 3 a.m. As we got back to our station and as I'm lying in bed, I can hardly believe what had occurred just a few short minutes ago. Every step that was required in order to save this lady's life was done by EMS personnel in the emergency room in front of a staff that should be treating the sniffles at some walk-in clinic.

I honestly can't say the lady would have died without the two of us at her side, but I do know, that treatment for her cardiac arrest would have been delayed unnecessarily.

The irony is that this is the same emergency room where Corporal Candy Ass is the "Director of Emergency Services". I find that fact highly entertaining.

Chapter 11
CATEGORY 5

In all of the years of my EMS career, there have been many extraordinary experiences. When it comes to career choices, there are few things that are comparable to the United States emergency services. The triad of police, fire, and EMS offers life experiences like no other. As an EMS provider, I've seen many things that range from the everyday mundane to the hypercritical patient who is teetering on death's doorstep.

In this range, a wide spectrum of comparisons can be made for car accidents. Like hurricanes, there are certain levels of severity of car accidents in accordance with the destruction and injury that is sustained. For example, a Category 1 hurricane is defined by winds between 74 and 95 miles an hour. You can make the argument that a Category 1 car accident may be little more than a fender bender and someone sustaining a couple of bruises or some such thing.

When it comes to a Category 5 hurricane, the winds have reached a minimum of 156 miles an hour. According to the experts, a Category 5 hurricane is as bad as it gets. Apparently, it doesn't matter whether the wind speed is 166, 176, or 186 miles an hour. I suppose when you consider the wind, rain, and tidal surge, and all of the destruction that it causes, I would conclude that the additional wind speed just doesn't matter much.

The same can be said for high-speed vehicular accidents. If you collide with another vehicle at 75, 85 or 95 miles an hour, the chances of survival are probably about the same—a little bit better than zero. The idea of categorizing traffic accidents like categorizing hurricanes is certainly not an official designation. People who work in law enforcement or better yet, in EMS probably know what a Category 5 accident would be. It is the type of accident that results in property obliteration and personal annihilation that simply doesn't get any worse than what you are looking at.

For example, is it really going to matter to the occupants of a car whether the car hits a tree or bridge support at 70, 80, or even 90 miles an hour? I think not. Ninety-nine times out of 100, I think all involved would be just as injured or just as dead. A motorcycle hits a car head-on and is obliterated and you are there picking up a dismembered and ripped up sack of broken bones that used to resemble a human body.

Another time, a car collides with a semi-tractor and trailer so hard that the car knocks the axle and steering wheels out from the cab of the truck. The car has disintegrated to the point that it is difficult to make out what color the car was and although you find the driver; you notice that most of his head is missing.

Or, it's the time a pick-up truck slams into a solid concrete bridge support so fast, and so hard, that you can't know for certain that there isn't someone else still trapped in the crushed and mangled wreckage. I would consider all of the above, Category 5.

One September weekend, our area received more than a foot of rain in a three-day period. Late Friday night and early Saturday morning, in the rain, my partner Brian Patterson and I were awakened at around 2:30 a.m. about a possible intentional drug overdose. When we arrived the local and county police departments were already on the scene. We were met by a police officer who said the woman who lived there might have overdosed in an attempt at suicide. When we found the patient she informed us that she was dying of lung cancer. She said that she had gotten into an argument with her sister. Apparently, during the course of yelling and screaming at each other, our patient's sister thought that she had taken an intentional overdose of prescription painkillers.

As we assessed her general physical condition, as well as her emotional and psychological status and counted the number pills or caplets she had remaining, we were able to discount any notion of a suicide attempt by way of a prescription drug overdose. We further consulted with the police department personnel present, and came to the conclusion that she most likely hadn't overdosed herself. Since it was the woman's sister and not her who called 9-1-1, she had very little intention of allowing us take her to the hospital without raising all kinds of hell.

Just as we were making the decision whether our reluctant patient was going to be put into police custody and transported to the nearest hospital, one of the officers in the house said, "A call came in for a single car accident. Your dispatcher wants to know if you are going to be able to respond to it."

I told the police officer in charge that due to finding nothing wrong with the lady and since she did not at all appear suicidal that I, for one, could not in good conscience ask the officers to put her into police protective custody. Therefore, he could relay to our dispatcher that Brian and I would be done here.

After briefly discussing her issues further with her, her sister's concerns about her supposed overdose and discovering no evidence of drug abuse or misuse, I was content to leave her at her home. The officers agreed with my decision and within a minute or two, Brian and I headed to the location of where it was reported that a car had slammed into a tree at a high rate of speed.

As the two of us got back into our ambulance, we quickly notified our dispatcher that we were clear of the previous call and headed toward the accident. It was at that time when we were first told that the police were there and they were announcing that they had two victims. One was a "K" (killed) and one was badly injured and the local fire department had been dispatched for extrication.

Even on rain-slicked roads, it only took us five minutes to arrive. Once we rolled up and came to a stop, I saw the Lincoln Township firefighters organizing and making ready their extrication equipment including the "Jaws of Life." (I found out later that they had only been on scene about five minutes before Brian and I arrived.) Several police officers were also on the scene including one officer who had been with us on our previous call.

As I exited the ambulance I immediately saw one of my Medic 1 colleagues working as one of the members of this particular local township fire department.

I shouted out to him over the roar of the fire trucks, "Anthony, what do you have here?"

He turned and yelled back, "The driver is a K and the other guy is half out of the car. His leg is pinned and he's basically unconscious!"

I raised my hand in acknowledgement and headed toward the car. I thought to myself, I'll start off by double-checking the status of the driver, just to make certain that he is in fact a fatality. After doing that, my concern, as well as the concerns of all of the other rescuers that have assembled themselves here tonight, can be with just one patient. All of us would singularly concentrate on the one task of removing and giving emergency medical treatment to the lone survivor of this Category 5 car wreck.

I approached the car and found it to have hit a tree that was more than three feet in diameter. The impact zone of the car was totally in the front end. By the way the car was crushed and wrapped around the tree it must have hit the tree at a tremendous speed. We learned that the car that contained the two 19-year old men started skidding on rain slicked roads at 87 miles an hour. The car skidded approximately one second before impacting the tree at 76 miles and hour. The "black-box" that this car contained, indicated that the car went from a speed of 76 miles an hour to zero in .02 seconds. That's less time than it takes to blink your eyes.

As I got to within ten feet of the car, I could see that there were several firefighters with extrication equipment and police officers holding flashlights around the passenger side of the car. Amongst and between their legs, I could see the body of a young man who had apparently been sitting on the front passenger seat, and was now laying half in and half out of the car.

I continued walking around to the back of the car and while approaching the driver's side, I could hear the firefighters starting their attempts to free the passenger who was a victim of this horrendous accident. Trying not to slip and fall on the loose soil and wet grass next to the driver's door, I used my flashlight to quickly visualize and assess the driver.

I found the driver to be crushed in a spot behind the steering wheel that was not survivable. From the edge of the dashboard that is in front of the steering wheel to the back of the front seat, it was no more than eighteen inches. From the distance of three feet, he looked dead.

As I reached for his neck, I could feel no pulse and his skin was a pale, milky white. Not surprisingly, he already started to feel colder than what would otherwise be considered normal. The last thing I did was to look into his eyes. The pupils of the eyes were dilated and non-reactive and had already started to glaze. There was no sign of life. The 19-year-old driver was dead and the victim of a self-inflicted tragedy.

In my mind, the driver (now) was a non-entity. From that moment forward, he didn't exist. My attention and singular focus and purpose would be what everyone else's had already moved to; to do the very best to free, render emergency medical treatment and transport the one and only patient of this "Category 5" accident.

As I quickly spun around and hustled to the passenger door, the door was already gone. Since the firefighters hadn't had time to remove the door, I believe the door was blown off of the car on impact. I quickly re-assessed the only patient we had and found him to be suffering from several different injuries.

He was principally unconscious, but not comatose. He was basically lying on his back on the ground in the mud and rain just outside the passenger door opening. He was flailing his arms and groaning, not aware of his surroundings or circumstances. It was his left leg that was holding him to the car and making it impossible for EMS and the firefighters assembled to remove him immediately.

During the tremendous impact, the cars motor and engine block was thrust into the passenger compartment carrying the dashboard and fire wall with it, instantly killing the teen-aged driver. The entire front end of the car was in what used to be the passenger compartment area. As we saw it, our patient had his leg most likely crushed up under the motor, which was smashed tightly between the tree and the rest of the car.

It was easy to see that our patient had a huge open fracture to his trapped leg that extended from just below the knee to more than half way to his ankle. The proximal tibia (part of the shinbone that is between the knee and the fracture site) was sticking through the gaping hole in the front of his leg, as was the distal (between ankle and the fracture site) tibia sticking upward. A large mid-portion of the bone itself was lying in pieces on what was left of the floorboard of the car.

It became obvious that he had broken both femurs (thigh bones). Although he had loose fitting clothes, I could see that anatomically speaking, his pelvis appeared asymmetrical. The easy conclusion is that more than likely he had sustained hip or pelvic fractures. On top of all of that, he had many lacerations to his face, hands and arms. It became instantly obvious that we were dealing with a highly unstable, critical patient that in all likelihood had incurred a multi-systems traumatic injury that involved the neurological, cardiovascular, musculoskeletal and possibly the respiratory operations of the body.

Up to this point Brian and I had been on the scene of this Category 5 accident for no more than five minutes. About that time, another ambulance from our company had arrived. When the original call was put out, it was reported that there would be two badly injured patients. Since there is no way to adequately treat two highly, unstable critical patients in the back of one ambulance, the second ambulance was dispatched to back us up in the event we had two patients. I don't care how talented a paramedic thinks they may be, when presented with two highly critical patients, you need two ambulances.

Bob White a paramedic, and Jamie Stone an EMT specialist, were now there to lend assistance to the only patient we were to have this night. I quickly updated the two of them as to the physical condition, apparent injuries and the task at hand of freeing our patient. During this time I had my partner record a set of vital signs for a part of the patient's general assessment as well as a baseline comparison for when the firefighters would set him free of the wreckage. As he was doing that, I turned my attention to assisting the firefighters in their efforts of extricating the lone survivor of this accident.

The first tool used to attempt to move, push or pry away the engine block from our patient's leg was the preeminent tool for vehicular extrication called the Jaws of Life. As a result of this particular head-on collision, the inside of the car was a pulverized, loosely held together, barely intact, piece of junk. Consequently, the effort to extricate our teen-aged patient resulted in just pushing around loose metal and plastic. The extrication effort utilizing the Jaws of Life was not able to move the engine block off of our patient's crushed leg and therefore free our patient.

The rescuers then tried another hydraulic tool. This one was a scissors looking device that is used to cut the posts on either side of the windshields of cars. This night it was utilized in an attempt to try to bite, cut or free the wreckage that might facilitate moving the motor off of our patient's leg. Again, no movement of the engine block.

Next up was a telescoping looking device that is used to spread objects apart. We pushed the engine block against the base of the seats our patient and victim had been sitting on. We pushed against the floor of the car. We pushed against the door posts. Ultimately, we failed in all of the many attempts to push the engine block off of our patient's leg.

The problem remained; there was nothing solid enough to push against that would enable the movement of the engine block. After more than twenty-five minutes and the use of the Jaws of Life, the scissors tool and two different sizes of spreading devices, we were no further ahead in freeing our patient. Although all of the firefighters were putting forth their best efforts, the rescue efforts were ineffective. Worse yet, the patient's vital signs were starting to deteriorate.

As the firefighters were trying the second size of the telescoping looking apparatus, my partner was now laying in the mud along side our patient with an IV in hand. At first I was just a little puzzled. Although on paper the idea is good to start an IV on a trapped victim of a car wreck, the first thing that usually happens is that the IV bag and the tubing get in the way of the rescuers efforts.

Secondly, you will invariably be infusing progressively colder and colder fluid into the blood stream. So unless it is absolutely necessary, I usually defer intravenous access until the victim has been freed and is inside a climate-controlled ambulance.

So I yelled out over all of the noise of this controlled chaos that we're involved with and said, "Brian, what are you doing? If that's not really, really necessary, let's forego that IV until we get him out of here!"

Brian looks up at me from the mud and rain and said, "His (blood) pressure is down to 70 systolic!"

That declaration raised an eyebrow.

"Okay, okay, do what you can." I responded.

Also by this time Bob, one of the other paramedics had gotten a non-rebreather oxygen mask around the patient's head and onto his face. But just about as fast as the mask touched his face, our disoriented patient was pulling it off. Bob and his partner Jamie tried several times before it became apparent that it also was a fruitless attempt at any sort of meaningful first-aid.

Just as Bob was pulling away the oxygen mask and bottle from our patient's face, Brian kneeled and was lying in the mud along with a police officer in an attempt to start an IV. The patient's arms were flailing and Brian's attempt to bolster our patient's blood pressure by infusing fluid into his compromised and rapidly depleting circulatory system was eventually unsuccessful. I was thinking that if the IV were in place, it could possibly buy us all a little more time in order to free him from the wreckage.

As I stood up and quickly assessed our lack of progress along with the rapidly deteriorating condition of our patient, I thought for perhaps the first time in my career about the real possibility of performing a field amputation. As Anthony, (being one of the finer paramedics at Medic 1), and I were briefly discussing the lack of progress and our growing frustration with this whole ordeal, I quickly turned to him and said, "Anthony, I'll be right back. I have to make a phone call."

I hustled over to where my ambulance was parked, jumped into the patient compartment and reached for the unit's cell phone. I dialed our hospital-based medical control to talk with the physician currently working in the emergency room. Dr. Clark answered.

I somberly said, "Dr. Clark, this is Jim from Medic. Listen, I'm at the scene of a really bad accident. A car has slammed into a tree at a really high rate of speed. The driver is dead and the only passenger is a teenage male who has his left leg pinned beneath the car motor. The firefighters have been working feverishly for more than thirty minutes and we haven't moved the motor an inch from his leg.

"This kid looks to me as though he is really starting to fade fast. He's got a head injury for sure; probable pelvic injuries; both femurs are broken and his left leg, just below the knee is just a mess. He has a comminuted (in several pieces) open fracture of the tibia of that same leg. I'm afraid that unless we can free him soon, we'll be extricating a body. So I'm calling you to tell you that I may have to take his leg off about three to four inches below the knee in order to get him out before he dies."

After more than thirty years of EMS experience, I'd seen all sorts of legs, arms and heads mangled, along with body parts and limbs being dismembered by being ripped or torn off and by being severed. I'd never had to do it myself. I've never been in the position where time was absolutely critical and rescue efforts despite all the hard work and sweat was so ineffective. I didn't know whether the good doctor was going to attempt to give some rudimentary advice on this or that. Or that he might say, "watch out for this or watch out for that."

I even thought that he might try to get a surgeon out to our accident scene to do the amputation. The truth is I just didn't know what to expect.

What I heard was, "Well Jim, I trust your judgment. Do the best you can and let us know what happens."

That was all he said.

At that moment, I felt strangely alone. I knew I was about to delve into unknown territory. Fortunately, I had thought years and years ago about what I would do if ever faced with such a dilemma. I had decided I would open one of our obstetrical kits and remove and use the scalpel from it. I knew that it would be new, sharp and sterile.

As I exited the ambulance and before I reached for the O.B. Kit, I told Anthony, "You've got just five minutes to get him the hell out of there. I've talked to the hospital already and I advised them on the whole situation and that more than likely, we were going to have to do a field amputation!"

Anthony kind of squinted at me like he wasn't sure what I had exactly said.

"Alright Jim, I'll see what I can do."

He spun around and started to walk briskly to where his fellow rescuers were doing their very best to trying again and again to free our dying patient. They were using every tool at their disposal and none of it seemed to be working.

Just as Anthony spun around, I turned and headed back to the ambulance. As I entered the patient compartment, I reached for the plexi-glass doors of the cabinet to where we kept the OB. Kits. I grabbed one, placed it on the bench seat and ripped it open. There was the scalpel, in its own sterile wrapper. I grabbed it from the kit and stuck it in the back pocket of my pants.

As I exited the ambulance I just stood back from a distance of no more than twenty feet and looked at the whole scene. I looked with grim intensity at the many people with their stern, rain, and sweat soaked faces. I watched them grimace and strain against the hard physical struggle of holding, pushing, and prying the heavy extrication equipment against a barely recognizable car that now was little more than a pile of plastic, rubber, and metal.

I observed the emotional stresses of firefighters in fruitless labor that was giving way to frustration in their countless and unsuccessful attempts to free this young man. I witnessed and shared the concern of my EMT and paramedic colleagues who tried and did ultimately fall short on starting the life sustaining IV. The position of our patient, his movement and flailing, the mud, the rain, and the darkness that was only interrupted by aerial lighting from the fire trucks, as well as the flashlights of the many police officers present, made it impossible to do anything that would be truly effective.

As I waited, I thought more and more about removing this kid's leg. I knew at that time that although it was the very last thing I wanted to do, I had best get my mind right for this most unenviable task. As the struggle to free our teenaged patient continued, I finally approached Anthony.

As I stood at his side, I said, "Well, are we any further along at all?"

Still working with his fellow firefighters, Anthony just turned to me and said, "No. Not really."

Although I had hoped that it would be different, I knew that unless we could quickly get a tow truck to pull the car from off of the tree, our extrication efforts in the end would be unsuccessful.

After a big sigh, I yelled out to Brian, "Get me another (blood) pressure!"

At the same time I motioned for Bob to join Anthony and me. Once Bob relinquished trying to keep a non-rebreather mask on our patient's face, he got up out of the dirt and mud and joined the two of us.

I said, "Okay, listen guys, I just talked to Dr. Clark in the E.R. and told him of the real possibility of having to take this kid's leg off."

Bob looked understandably a little surprised and said, "What did he say to that?"

I responded by repeating word for word what he told me.

Just as I finished telling Bob about the very limited words of wisdom coming from the E.R., Brian yelled out, "Stine, his pressure is now 60 systolic!"

That was it. At that moment I knew we could either extricate a young man with one leg alive, or we could eventually remove a whole, lifeless body. In that context the decision seemed easy for me.

With all of that in mind and the patient's blood pressure falling like a stone I announced to my two colleagues, "Listen guys, we're going to have to take his leg off right now."

Anthony was still working in vain and directing the continuing efforts to free our patient, but I knew he was listening to me.

It was then that I looked at Bob and said in an uneasy tone, "Listen, I know that I'm as arrogant as it gets, but this is even ballsy for me! Does anybody have a better idea?"

Bob turned to me and said, "I don't, and nothing we've done so far has worked."

Anthony said, "Jim, do what you have to do."

That was the final verdict. At the time I was really glad and immensely relieved that Bob and Anthony were there. The whole idea would have been all the more difficult to do had I not had two other experienced and highly-respected paramedics with me at the scene of this terrible and tragic accident.

I told Anthony that he could tell the firefighters to stand down with their efforts.

With that I approached Brian and said "Patterson, we're going to take his leg off and get him out of there right now."
Brian looked up at me from the patient's side and from the look on his face I could tell that he was a little shocked at my declaration of intent. Seeing the look of, "we're going into unknown territory here!" I quickly responded by saying, "Brian, we don't have a choice. He's probably going to die anyway, but if we don't get him out now and to the hospital, he's going to die for sure!"

"Do you want to get a tourniquet around his leg first?" was the only thing he said.

With that, I knew at that moment his thinking had shifted from whether we should, to how we could.

In response to his tourniquet question, I thought at first that due to the severity of our patient's traumatic injuries that his body would be shunting the blood away from his extremities and to his vital organs and because of that his leg really by this time would not be bleeding much at all. But nonetheless, it wasn't a bad idea.

"Okay, let's do that. Bob, can you find a triangular bandage and get it out of our unit?"   Bob was off in a brisk walk and was back within a minute with ace wraps and stating that he couldn't find the triangular bandages.

I said back to him, "I don't think that's going to work. Hold on for a second."

With that, I popped my personal pager off of my belt and stuck it in my pocket. I quickly un-cinched my belt, pulled it through the belt loops and handed my belt to Bob.

"Here Bob, use this. Just wrap it as tightly as you can just above his knee."

Bob didn't say a word, he just promptly did what I asked and had it extremely tight around his lower thigh. As he was doing that, I was calling out to the many police officers on the scene, "I need some more light here!"

Bob's partner that night, Jamie Stone, informed me that she had removed the ambulance cot and had it next to the car and that if we needed more bandages to control the possibility of additional hemorrhage, she was ready to assist Bob and me.

A couple of the firefighters that just a few short minutes ago were giving their best efforts with the many different pieces of extrication, were now down in the mud and slop with my partner Brian. They were there to help keep our patient as still as possible and to swiftly slide him out from under the wreckage once he was free.

In a matter of a short few seconds, two police officers were shining their lights into the wreckage of the car. I reached into my back pocket and pulled out the wrapper that contained the scalpel. I removed the wrapper and the guard that was protecting the blade. I put the scalpel down toward the young man's leg and decided to cut from the posterior aspect (back of the leg) rather than where the leg was already badly injured.

Without looking at my good friend and colleague, I simply said in a somewhat soft voice, "Bob help me roll his leg over, if you can."

As we rolled it over, the back of our patient's leg didn't have a single mark on it. It was absolutely pristine. I called down to Brian and Jamie and said, "Brian, you guys hold him still! Bob is going to me help me by holding his thigh as best as he can."

While I'm telling my two colleagues to hold our patient motionless,

I'm thinking that as far as his impending amputation is concerned, I'm glad that he is essentially unconscious. If he hadn't been, I would have to sedate him as best as I could and still work through the screams of agony that would surely follow such a procedure. I turned to the two or three police officers who were holding flashlights and pointed to the exact spot of where the incision would be made.

"Guys, I need the light directed onto the back of our patient's leg right here." I looked at Bob and said, "Okay, let's do this."

With that I took the scalpel in my left hand, held his leg just below the knee with my right hand, poked the skin with the tip of the scalpel blade, and inserted it about a half inch. As I pulled the handle of the blade in a downward motion, I was struck by how easily the blade cut through the tissue.

With the first stroke of the scalpel, the skin instantly parted and since the incision site was snowy white, I knew I had cut past both layers of skin and into the fatty tissue. Since this was the first time I had ever done such a thing as this, I was surprised just how wide the skin retracted. Being fully aware of the elasticity of human skin, and especially that of young adults, I was still surprised to see the skin retract a good three inches. The next stroke of the scalpel brought me into the outer portion of the calf muscle. The next several strokes brought me deeper and deeper into this young man's muscular leg. The one thing I tried to do was to stay totally focused and concentrate so as to cut deeper into the exact same spot. My thought was that if I could do that, I would not remove muscle tissue by segmenting it in different spots. Even with those thoughts and trying to stay focused with the task at hand, I felt more and more uncomfortable with each and every stroke of the scalpel.

The worst part was that, although I knew what had to be done and must be done, a small part of me felt like I was further injuring and mutilating a young man who was already critically injured and who above all didn't need another injury. Even as uncomfortable as I felt, I was extremely confident that my actions along with those of my colleagues were at this time without question, completely right and absolutely necessary.

As I was cutting, I yelled to Brian and Jamie, "After we get him free, keep the end of his leg out of the mud!"

After perhaps as many as a dozen or more strokes of the scalpel I had encountered the fibula (small bone it the leg). I was completely surprised and caught off guard when I found the fibula to be intact. I thought for sure that as crushed and broken into pieces that the tibia was, that the fibula too, would be in the same condition.

Although the fibula is basically in the middle of the leg and surrounded by heavy muscle masses, I was just sure that in all probability, the fibula would be fractured as well. Much to my chagrin, that wasn't the case. It was bad enough that I had to cut this young man's leg off, now I had to break a bone in his leg as well.

I first tried to break the bone with my fingers but due to the thickness of the calf muscle, I was unable to get any kind of leverage to do so. I then tried to use the scalpel as a saw and attempted to cut into the bone. That didn't work.

Bob immediately retrieved a knife from his pants pocket—one of those paramilitary type knives with a razor sharp, serrated edge that are fairly common. He opened it, and I exchanged with him my scalpel for his knife. Surprisingly, even with its serrated edge, that particular knife wouldn't cut through the bone either. With out asking, a firefighter who apparently was watching this ordeal, handed me a wire cutter. As I took it from him, I was sincerely hoping that this would do the trick. It did. It took four cuts from the wire cutter to sever the small bone. I then handed the wire cutter to one of the police officers present and Bob handed my scalpel back to me. Three or four cuts later I had fully severed our patient's leg.

"Alright Brian, he's free. Get him out of here!"

As quickly as I said that, Brian, Jamie, and a couple of firefighters were pulling him onto the backboard they had placed under his head and shoulders. With a cervical collar already in place, our patient was finally being extricated from the wreckage. He was quickly slid onto the backboard but the only thing I asked them to do was not to let his severed leg get into the mud.

Just as he was being moved his leg fell into the dirt and mud. I couldn't believe it.

"Get his leg up! Get it out of the damn mud!" I yelled. Immediately Brian grabbed our patient's leg and raised it while the other two firefighters continued to drag our patient and secured him to the backboard. I was up to my elbows in blood and I needed to change my gloves. No sooner did I exchange my blood soaked gloves for clean ones, than the ambulance cot carrying our patient was being slid into the back of the ambulance.

I yelled out a very appreciative and heart felt "thank-you" to the firefighters and without delay started to reassess our patient. As critical as he was, I asked Bob to ride in with me as Brian drove. I needed Bob to start a large bore IV for me while I evaluated his vital signs including possible advanced airway management. If his breathing was the slightest bit compromised, I would have to intubate our patient to ensure a patent and protected airway and if needed I could add oxygen too.

Other than the obvious head injury, the field amputated leg and his bilateral femur and possible pelvic fractures I now noticed that our patient was trying to brush aside our oxygen mask. I then yelled out to Brian that we were ready to go. Bob started a second IV while I continuously evaluated and treat our patient. I had just finished placing the electrodes on our patient's chest to monitor his heart rate and rhythm and was busy listening to his lung sounds when I noticed the crevices of the mattress of the ambulance cot was starting to fill up with blood to the point that it was just oozing around the edges of the top of our backboard.

Bob had just completed starting the IV and as I jerked the stethoscope out of my ears, I asked him, "Bob, where in the hell is all of this blood coming from?"

I looked at our patient's severed leg and that wasn't bleeding to any degree of concern. Although he had several lacerations to his head, face and arms the life sustaining blood that was now on our cot far outweighed anything that was obvious.

I continued, "Bob, there is something really wrong here. Cut his clothes off! Cut all of his damn clothes off!"

By this time he had been in our ambulance for less than two minutes when I realized that there was going to be something awfully bad when we were able to see his whole body. Unfortunately, I wasn't wrong.

I was sitting on a cushioned seat at the head of the patient, and Bob was sitting on the bench seat and to the patient's left side, as he lay supine on our ambulance cot. Without delay we started cutting clothes. Our patient had a pair of jogging type pants on and a T-shirt. Bob started cutting from the bottom of the pant leg and was going up and I started at the top of his T-shirt and was cutting downward. As I was cutting, a whole cluster of things crossed my mind.

"Did he have a chest wound?" I didn't think so only because for all of the time he was on the ground, he never was in any kind of respiratory distress. Besides, his lung sounds were reasonably clear. "Did he have an abdominal wound?" Could be, but his belly was not rigid or hard or anything that would resemble internal bleeding.

Furthermore, that's internal not external, and it quickly became obvious there was some major hemorrhaging going on from somewhere. Then I thought, "What about rectal bleeding? It's pretty much the only thing left."

As Bob continued cutting I was still trying to keep the oxygen mask on his face and our patient was just as busy pulling it off. Finally, I just duct taped his wrist to our cot side rails. Just as Bob cut his underwear off of him, both of us had a collective gasp and groan. The patient had a huge laceration that was perhaps five inches in length in his perineum. For the male patient, that's between the scrotum and the anus. It was a diagonal laceration that was long and apparently very deep.

Blood was pouring out onto our cot at such a rate that I instantly became alarmed that our patient could pump out his remaining blood volume within the next few minutes.

"Brian, let's move!" I screamed as Brian drove as fast as he could, sirens blaring and lights flashing. "We've got to get to the hospital now!"

I could feel the ambulance accelerate. Brian did a good job by hollering back to Bob and me when he was coming to railroad crossings, sharp turns, breaking for lights and traffic.
At the same time I was yelling for Brian to "put his foot in it" as Bob reached for the trauma dressings; the biggest bandages that EMS carries. They measure 12" X 30" inches and we used all of the six that we normally carry.

I hit the button on our cardiac monitor that records blood pressure and Bob flipped open the roller clamp on the IV tubing to wide open, so we could infuse our patient with more fluid. Then the both of us got exceedingly aggressive with attempting to control his hemorrhaging. His blood pressure was just under fifty systolic and getting him to the hospital alive was now suddenly in question.

But Bob and I did our very best to pack and hold pressure to the gaping wound. We soaked within five minutes all of our trauma dressings. It was unbelievable the amount of blood that was being pumped from his vascular system. I told Bob that had I known just how badly he was bleeding I would have taken his leg off earlier. Bob agreed.

Again I changed gloves. This time I had to relinquish them in order to call the emergency room and so as not to contaminate our communication equipment. I advised the staff there that we did indeed have to do the field amputation that I had discussed with the emergency room doctor earlier, but now we felt that his most critical wound wasn't from his leg or face or head, but from his pelvis. Bob and I were now certain that something had lacerated his perineum, but had also somehow lacerated some of the pelvic arteries or veins. I relayed our findings and thoughts on what we believed his injuries were to the emergency room personnel so the staff was ready when we arrived.

As we rolled to a stop in the ambulance parking area of the emergency room approximately ten minutes after we departed from the accident site, there were several nurses and hospital employed EMT's awaiting our arrival at the entry point to the emergency room. They assisted Bob, Brian and me in taking our patient to one of the large trauma rooms. Once there, I further updated our patient's condition and our findings since I had last talked with them five to six minutes before our arrival. It's amazing what can change in a critical patient's status in that little amount of time.

I told the staff that although it was an easy clinical observation that our patient had a head injury and although he had a leg and a half instead of two legs that neither of those issues could cause his death. I told the attending doctor, "…that if anything kills this kid it will be his pelvic injuries." The awful fact of the matter was that without immediate emergency surgery, there would be no way to replace the blood at the rate his body was loosing it.

The call had already been put into the on-call trauma surgeon who is responsible for this type of thing. As he arrived, he asked me what and how things had happened. He wanted to know what the circumstances were with the mechanics of the accident, time spent on scene, emergency treatment rendered prior to our arrival to the hospital and so forth.

As the surgeon was listening to me relate all of the information that he requested, he is doing a physical exam on our patient. What he found was astonishing. What had apparently happened was that the pelvic injury occurred from flying debris during the high-speed deceleration. The surgeon reached up into the patient's pelvis through the laceration in his perineum. He in fact had most of his hand inside the patient and pulled out at least three large pieces of a CD.

Somehow a CD went airborne upon impacting the tree and flew through the air, cutting his jogging pants, lacerating the perineum, ripping and cutting organs and tissue deep into the patient's pelvic cavity. The x-rays showed that his pelvis was just a mess. Bilateral femur fractures and fractures to the pelvis and fluid in the abdominal cavity were readily apparent.

When you stack all of that on top of an amputated limb and a head injury, the patient we delivered to the local emergency room was too much to deal with by the on-call surgeon. After several units of blood were infused and an extensive patient evaluation was performed the decision was made to transport our patient to a regional trauma center.

But, with all of the rain that had fallen and continued to fall, the trauma center's helicopter was not flying. That left the job of transporting our patient by way of ground transport. Once the decision was made to transfer our patient nearly sixty miles to the regional trauma center, it was just a matter of making sure our patient was stable enough for the trip.

The two paramedics who were assigned to do the emergency transfer were extremely uncomfortable with the severity of the injuries and the uncertainty of the survival of our patient. This led to the decision of Medic 1 not do the transfer without the trauma surgeon accompanying the patient. After almost three hours of treatment in the local emergency room, our patient was being transferred with two highly qualified and experienced paramedics, the trauma surgeon and a veteran emergency room nurse. An hour later, the patient was at the trauma center in Kalamazoo.

Unfortunately, all of the dozens of people who came to the assistance to our patient including MFR's, EMT's, paramedics, doctors, nurses, surgeons and the resources of two hospitals, it was not enough to save the life of our patient. He succumbed to his injuries approximately nine hours after the tragic accident.

The name of my patient that night was Zachary Schoenbach. I knew that before we had left the scene of the accident. From his body build I suspected that he had been a high school athlete. I was right about that. What I didn't know about Zach was that he had been a high school wrestler. He also had interests in playing basketball, skate boarding and BMX stunt bike riding. He was a young man who was gainfully employed and still enjoyed life to the fullest.

It would be fair to say Zach was much like most athletic, young men. He worked hard, played hard and partied hard. He just made a mistake by drinking and then climbing into a car with a friend who had made the same error. Zach's mother told me that her son had an interest in pursuing a career in mechanical engineering and wonders if he would have continued with his schooling. She thinks of him often, every day and for a short time after his death, doubted whether she could go on without him.

She carries at least a half dozen pictures of her beloved son in her wallet and recalls with reverence the particulars of each photo. She considers with a smile if he would have had a wife and family. His sister told me of the playful sibling rivalry they shared and how she still misses her brother.

Many people in the Lakeshore Public School District felt the loss of such a vibrant young man as Zach's wrestling coach gave a heartfelt and moving eulogy during Zach's funeral. His many friends left roadside flowers, messages and memorials at the scene of the accident.

The saddest for me is the regrets that Zach's family and friends will forever have. It is the irreplaceable thought of what might have been.

Chapter 12
AGGIE AND HERBIE: A LOVE STORY

If you are in this business for any length of time at all, you will run into many unique individuals, couples, or personalities. Once in a great while, you might run into all three in one place and time. Such is the case of Aggie and Herbie. Together they were one of the wildest, and ill-suited couples I have ever seen. But, it was their clashing personalities that on dozens of occasions lent to some of the funniest EMS moments of my career.

With all of their bumbling and blundering, the two of them really reminded me of the old comedy duo of Laurel and Hardy. When I first started my employment at Medic 1, they were in their late 30s or early 40s. Herbie was a little bitty guy who was a big time boozer. When he was sober enough to stand up straight, he was perhaps five-feet eight inches tall and maybe at best 130 pounds. Whenever I saw Herbie he was invariably well intoxicated with the cheapest "rot-gut" wine he could find. Even though he was perpetually drunk and exhibited a lot of false bravado, essentially he was harmless.

Aggie, on the other hand, was just about the polar opposite of Herbie. Aggie was about six feet tall and was a dozen donuts shy of 450 pounds. She was a type II diabetic who usually ignored her disease and failed to take care of her health. She also had a bad temper and a mean streak a mile long that Herbie found himself on the wrong side of on many occasions. I don't recall her ever being outwardly drunk, but she was always as mad as hell at something or someone. More times than not, that certain someone, was little 'ole Herbie. But, for better or for worse, they were usually together.

I don't know how they treated each other during the "good times," but I did see and witnessed the wreckage left behind during the bad times. Of course, neither of them ever showed that they had more than ten minutes of formal education and it was always terribly obvious that neither of them found themselves too close to a bar of soap and a bath tub. This is why so many of us at Medic 1 found them so aggravating and at the same time, incredibly entertaining.

The first time I met Herbie and Aggie, was more than thirty years ago. It was a cold, overcast, and blustery November day with a frosty wind and a few snowflakes flying around. There was just enough snow on the ground to collect in small corners and crevices on the street. At that time I was working with an EMT by the name of Dave Hawkins. We had just finished running a call and were just leaving the hospital when we got dispatched for injuries from a domestic violence incident.

We acknowledged the dispatch and inquired whether the police were en route. With this type of call and the emotions it generates, it can prove to be very dangerous for any kind of emergency service. Since it was the police who called us after receiving the call, they assured us they were on their way.

Two police cruisers were already at the house that looked like a dilapidated, rundown farm shack. About a third of its windows were broken or missing. The roof was in disrepair and it probably hadn't been painted in the fifty or more years since the old wooden house was first built. I stepped out of the ambulance wearing my winter coat, sock hat and carrying my trauma box.

The first thing I noticed was this little, skinny guy who had a few minor lacerations and dozens of heavy scratch marks all over his hands, arms, face, neck, and shoulders. He was wearing just a "wife-beater" T-shirt and a pair of pants. He was clearly mad at some woman, because he was muttering something about, "that big fat bitch."

He was walking around outside bare-foot in the cold, picking at what looked like thorns out of his arms. He didn't seem to be seriously injured, so I walked past him and into the house to meet an upset Aggie talking to one of the police officers. What I saw was a huge behemoth of a woman standing in the middle of a kitchen and living room area that appeared to just have had a hurricane go through it. The place was just a wreck. Broken plates, cups and dishes were everywhere. The few pieces of furniture they had in the house were either broken or tipped over.

She stood with an intense look of anger on her face. Her hair is a mess and she has what appears to be what remains of a dozen meals on the dress that she is wearing. I briefly turned my attention to the officer. He told me her name was Agatha.

Before I could acknowledge his answer, she yelled, "My name be

Aggie! Nothin' else, just Aggie!"

I looked at her, shrugged my shoulders and in a matter of fact tone said, "Okay, Aggie it is."

As I started to step toward her, she didn't look at me at all. She just kept her eyes fixed on the police officer. She clearly didn't care for either his line of questioning or attitude before I entered the room. Most assuredly she didn't like the officer calling her by her proper name.

After observing the results of a possible melee and looking her over for apparent injuries, the only thing I found was an approximately six-inch, full thickness laceration to the back of one of her massive thighs. With the fatty tissue exposed, her cut looked like a tablespoon full of large curd cottage cheese had spilled onto the side of a grain silo. By the look on her face she was much too angry to be aware of any pain that she might otherwise be feeling.

She reminded me of a boxer lightly dancing in their corner prior to the start of the bout, ready to spring out at the night's opponent. Instantly I could tell that this was nobody to mess with or to take lightly.

"I'm goin' to kill dat lil mothafucka one of dees days!" she said with promise in her voice.

She continually refused to quit moving around so I could properly bandage her wound and I was getting irritated.

"Do you want me to wrap this or not?" I said sternly. Without ever having met me, or for that matter ever having seen me before, she looked like she wanted to punch me in the face in the worst way.

"I don't give a fuck what you do, mothafucka!"

With that heartfelt statement, the police officer got in her face. He told her in no uncertain terms and in the language she was accustomed to, that any further talk like that would land her in jail. At about the same time, I hear some yelling and commotion going on outside. So without wrapping her wound, I walked back outside to see that the guy that had been picking thorns out of his arms was Aggie's boyfriend, Herbie.

It appeared to me that he was on the short end of a heated argument with the other of the two officers who had responded to the disturbance. Apparently this particular officer out of the goodness of his heart had given Herbie a winter coat about a month previous to the onset of the cold weather. He asked Herbie several times as to the whereabouts of the winter coat. Herbie was being evasive and the cop was getting more than a little pissed off.

"Where in the hell is that coat and why don't you have it on?" the officer said, demanding an answer.

After the cop really starts to go nose-to-nose with Herbie, the "Stan Laurel" routine came out. When the character, Laurel, was being scolded by Oliver Hardy, Laurel's lower lip would start quivering and he would get teary-eyed and he would start to whine and cry. Then he would tell Ollie, in that high squeaky voice, how sorry he was for screwing something up. Well that's what Herbie would do after being confronted by any authority figure.

So after a few minutes of whining and crying, Herbie finally came clean and admitted to the police officer that he had traded the coat for two bottles of the "good stuff." When the officer heard what had happened to his coat, he became so exasperated that I thought he might just shoot Herbie right then and there. When I saw and heard all of this, I immediately knew I had met a couple of real characters and I started to laugh my ass off. I couldn't help it. This was like a great comedy routine you would have to pay good money to see, unless you were on-duty as a paramedic or a police officer.

After chastising and scolding Herbie mightily for three or four minutes, we all walked back into the house. It was then that I noticed that it wasn't really any warmer inside than it was outside. As I looked around, I saw that the place was being heated by the kitchen stove and oven. There was a hole over the kitchen sink where the window used to be; a hole with a couple of pieces of rotted slats of wood hanging down from it. That hole was the result of one of their usual arguments turned violent, where they started throwing all kinds of dishes, cups, pots and pans at each other.

The kitchen area had been lit by a single strand of wire hanging from the kitchen ceiling with a solitary light bulb at the end of it. By the look and scope of the mess, it was of course to nobody's surprise that the light bulb was broken.

As the story goes–and from what each of the two lovers had to say to the cops– Aggie got a hold of Herbie, picked him up over her head and literally threw him over the kitchen sink and right through the window. If that wasn't bad enough, the reason Herbie was so scratched up when we had first arrived was because he had landed right into the middle of a large thorny bush that was just outside and under where the kitchen window used to be.

While he was busy extricating himself from the briars, Aggie found and climbed on top of this rickety old kitchen chair, carrying a new light bulb. As she is attempting to change the bulb, Herbie came back into the house to see her standing tall on the chair with her flabby arms extended high over her head. Without a second thought (or a first thought for that matter), he proceeded to kick the chair out from under her.

I know I may have a twisted sense of humor that not everybody may appreciate. But just the thought of her being launched off of that chair and landing on her ass, on the floor in a thunder clap, still to this day, makes me smile. She hit the broken glass and porcelain-covered floor with such force she received the laceration to the back of her thigh.

As Herbie, the police officer, and I walked through the front door, Aggie and Herbie saw each other and immediately resumed their yelling and attempting to get at each other. I wasn't surprised a bit when I noticed that Aggie was trying harder than her man. There was little doubt in my mind, that if they were left alone for just a minute, the fighting would have started all over again and Herbie would have most likely found himself being tossed through another window.

After they exchanged their heartfelt personal insults with an array of colorful vulgarity, the police officers at last separated the two of them into different rooms. This was done as much to get each of their stories as to what had happened to spark this particular fight, but mostly as it was to keep them from quite possibly and seriously hurting each other.

Aggie really needed to have her laceration stitched together. Unbeknownst to her, I suggested to one of the officers that we should force her to go to the hospital by threatening to take her to the county jail if she wouldn't allow us to take her. I told the officer that if we just wrapped it up and left her here that in about an hour after it started hurting real good, she would be calling us back for a ride anyway.

The officer agreed.

After my partner and I finished bandaging the still open wound, she did consent to have us take her to the local emergency room for further treatment. Of course that wasn't before she raised all kinds of hell about why it was that she might have to go to jail instead of "dat dirty lil basted ova dare!" Apparently it was lost on Aggie that it was she who happened to throw Herbie out of the house by way of the kitchen window.

We then fully assessed Herbie and found him to be essentially unhurt. I remember telling Herbie that if he took a bath and put on some clean clothes once in a while, he would be just fine. The two officers were satisfied with Herbie's rendition of what had transpired and why. Although I'm sure the two police officers didn't believe everything he had to say, they did decide to leave Herbie at the house.

Aggie, as overweight as she was, could walk, but it still took me and my partner three or four attempts and a lot of pushing and shoving to get her into the ambulance. I asked the officer whether he had met either of the two of them before today. He said that he had known them for as long as he was on the police department (which was not quite a year), and this type of complaint between the two of them was nothing new. He figured that if they could keep the two of them separated for three to four hours, they would both cool off and everything would be fine until the next time.

I too, would see the couple often in the years to come as a paramedic. I am sure that she broke his nose at least twice, not to mention the numerous times that there were scalp and facial lacerations, eyes that were swollen shut and lips that were noticeably fattened. She even stabbed him on one occasion and gave him a superficial wound to one of his shoulder blades.

There were two things you could always count on if Aggie had just worked over Herbie. The first is that Herbie would be as mad as hell at Aggie. We would always know he was going to be all right if he was yelling at the top of his lungs and calling her a "no good fat bitch!" or some other such pleasantry. As we would be wheeling Herbie out of their house and to our waiting ambulance, the other thing you could always count on would be Aggie just crying her eyes out. She would be telling Herbie (usually at the same time he is yelling at her), how much she loved him and how sorry she was. It was always quite the show and truly a sight to behold. In retrospect, I honestly do believe that she was genuinely sorry. I guess Aggie never got a handle on that anger management thing.

For whatever reason, the two of them would separate every now and again, and I would find Aggie living with her mother. As it turned out, she didn't get along with her mother appreciably better than she did with Herbie. Although there was always plenty of yelling, cussing and screaming between Aggie and her mother, I don't recall either of them ever beating the hell out of each other. It might be because that within fifty pounds, they were about the same size and shape.

Unlike the domestic violence calls that I received when Aggie and Herbie were together, the one reason (more than any other) an ambulance would be called when Aggie and her mother were together was for a perceived medical issue. Like Aggie, her mother was basically a non-compliant diabetic. That meant more times than not one of them would be a little disoriented and therefore unable to think or reason clearly. When this would happen to either Aggie or her mother, the arguing, yelling, and screaming would still be loud enough to hear from the street.

To make matters potentially worse, Aggie's mother resided in an old two-story house, which was divided into an upstairs and down-stairs apartment. Naturally, she lived in the upstairs apartment that was only accessible by a set of wooden stairs, which was constantly in a poor state of disrepair. Those steep, shabby steps were more hazardous during the winter months when they were perpetually covered with ice and snow.

When either of them wanted an ambulance, if they couldn't walk, they couldn't go. It was as simple as that. If an actual emergency had occurred in their apartment the local fire department would have been needed for some sort of aerial ladder or bucket extrication. Fortu-nately, that was never the case.

Another time when we were called to Aggie's house, was to help her out for an unknown problem. Although this complaint turned out to be extremely minor, it was highly unusual. As is usual, on this particu-lar day, we were really busy. Nonetheless, we were dispatched to a residence I happened to know all too well. I really wasn't in any mood to see her, and was mildly annoyed at the thought of having to listen to her song and dance as to why she needed an ambulance. But, she called for assistance and we are obligated to help if we can.

As a lack of luck would have it, we had a student nurse riding with us on this particular day. (In most nursing programs today, the student nurses are required as part of their training and education to ride with paramedics for two or three eight hour shifts.) It's not that I dislike student nurses or for that matter students of any kind, it's just when they are in my ambulance I'm responsible for their actions as well as their safety. It's just a big pain that I just as soon not have.

Over the years I've seen bunches of EMT, paramedic as well as nursing students as riders observing, learning and hopefully appreciating all of the facets of modern EMS. Most of those who think they want to get into this business, really don't know what they are getting into or why. After all, pre-hospital medicine is not at all the controlled atmosphere of the hospital emergency room setting. Even the most chaotic emergency room is much more controlled than any kind of "street medicine" setting.

My partner and I, along with the newly acquired female student nurse arrived at Aggie's house. After beating on the door and getting no answer, we walked around the house in knee-deep weeds and saw her through a window. She was sitting on the couch in her living room, watching TV and acting as though nothing was out of the ordinary. You would think if you had called an ambulance, you just might be concerned enough to at least watch for its arrival.

As I saw her sitting there and not answering the door, I was instantly aggravated. When she saw us, she got up, unlocked the door and let the three of us into the house.

As we walked into the kitchen area, I said to her, "What's the problem today Aggie?"

"I gots to go to da hospital," she proudly professed.

"I kind of figured that out, or you wouldn't have bothered us," I said as a matter of fact. "So what's the problem today as opposed to any other day?"

"It's my tooff, god damn it!"

"What do you mean it's your tooth? I snapped back, "You called an ambulance for your tooth?" I said, highly irritated.

Without the slightest thought of her misusing the ambulance service, she says, "I said I gots to get to the hospital, so day kin take care of my tooff."

"Just what is so wrong with your tooth that needs the services of an ambulance and a hospital?"

"Dis right here!"

She then proceeded to put her hands on her hips, leaned back slightly, and gave me a smile that only a Jack-O-Lantern would be proud of. She then pushed her tongue against her lower front teeth. Sure enough, she had a lower incisor that was moving quite freely as she pushed her tongue against it. She was able to move her tooth like a wobbling, spinning top. She then continued to tell the three of us that her tooth had been getting more loose over the last couple of days. Now, she wanted to use the ambulance as a taxi for transportation to the local hospital...so she could have it removed.

By now, I'm becoming more than a little aggravated at this whole idiotic call and admittedly a little embarrassed at having a student nurse see what we as EMS providers deal with.

I grabbed one of her kitchen chairs and I said to her, "Sit down on this chair and don't move."

I already had on my rubber gloves. So, as Aggie was getting comfortable on her chair, I reached into my pants pocket and pulled out a four-by-four inch gauze pad. I told her to lean her head back, way back, and to open her mouth. When she opened her pie hole, I noticed that she no longer had most of her teeth. The remaining few appeared to be in various stages of decay.

I grabbed hold of that slimy, brown, nasty tooth with the gauze pad and proceeded to twist and pull it back and forth. Although the tooth seemed ready to literally fall out, I found it difficult to extract. It was much more stable than what it first looked. It still needed to come out. It just didn't need to be done at the hospital. Nor did she need an ambulance ride to a hospital to have it pulled.

So here I am, trying to get a solid hold of this half rotted, slimy tooth and now she wants to talk to us.

As I kept pulling, pushing and twisting, I said to her, "No talking! You have a dentist at work here!"

Now of course, my partner, Scott is just laughing his head off. It was just a few seconds more and a few more twists and I pulled it right out of her mouth.

After I pulled it out, I said to my partner, "There; we're outta here!"

Aggie then jumped up and immediately started running her tongue back and forth across the latest hole in her head. She looked like a big, fat snake standing there with a stupid look on her face.

As she stood there doing her cobra routine, I said to her, "There ya' are Aggie. Good enough for you?"

"Good enough, ambulance driver," she said.

As the three of us walked out of her house, Scott just couldn't believe I pulled her tooth, root and all.

As we are just climbing back into our ambulance he said, "Stine, I can't believe you just did that!"

I just shrugged and simply said, "Well, it was just about ready to fall out anyway. We just saved the taxpayers a few bucks. On top of that, the nurses at the emergency room won't be mad at us for bringing her in."

I remember as I was busy pulling her tooth, I happened to glance at the student nurse who had been riding with us. I will never forget the look of bewilderment and shock on her face. She looked absolutely aghast with disbelief and stood there in stunned silence. All of that is because the student nurse is not and was not a member of EMS and as a result, was totally out of her element. Up to this point and time, part of her formal education in medicine did not prepare her for how things "can" be from time to time in some areas of our country. Her reaction was as funny as the call itself.

***

As the years rolled by, I saw Aggie and Herbie dozens of times. Probably one of the funniest things I ever did was to instigate a fight between them. I know what you're thinking. However, after you gasp and have a moment of apoplexy, consider this. Could I ever come into your house and within let's say, two minutes have you and your significant other fighting? The answer is: I don't think so! However, we're not talking about a couple of brain surgeons here. We're talking about two people who are in dire need of brain surgeons.

At this time we had a new employee at Medic 1 who was assigned to be my partner. His name was Dave Nelson. Although Dave was a new employee at this ambulance service, he was not new to the business. He's retired now, but in his day, he was a fine and talented paramedic with tons of experience and know how.

It was about midnight on a warm summer evening and we were sitting and watching TV at our central station in Benton Harbor. We received a dispatch to respond in a non-emergency status to Aggie and Herbie's house. The only thing the dispatcher knew, as far as the complaint was concerned was that "a woman is feeling ill."

I turned to Dave in a fit of glee and said, "Oh man, that's Aggie and Herbie's place... you've got to see this."

As we walked out to the ambulance, I could hardly contain myself. I told him that, "This is not an ambulance call. This is an event!" As I briefly told Dave about some of the antics of this odd couple, we both jumped into the ambulance and took a leisurely drive over to their house. As I pulled up into their short driveway, I hit the switch to activate our left-sided floodlights in order to illuminate the distance between our ambulance and their front door.

We got out of the rig, walked up to their front porch and proceeded to knock on the door. Herbie answered the door and as usual reeked with a combination of cheap wine, stale beer, rot gut whiskey, general body odor, and really bad breath.

"So Herbie, what's going on tonight?"

Before he can answer, Aggie spoke up from across the room, "I don't feel good."

"Okay Aggie, what do you mean you don't feel good?"

"I just don't feel right. I think I'm sick or something." she said, frowning to express her discomfort.

Dave checked her blood sugar and it was in the 400's, which is really very high. As usual, I admonished her for the umpteenth time about not taking care of her health. And for the umpteenth time, she didn't give a damn what I had to say about that or anything else for that matter, and told me as much.

I quickly winked at my partner and casually turned around to Aggie and said, "I'll bet you're not eating anything worthwhile, are you." I walked right past her and opened the refrigerator door. I looked inside and there was virtually nothing that appeared to be edible by anything this side of a goat or buzzard. I hollered at Herbie, "What in the hell does Aggie cook for you? This looks terrible!"

As anticipated, Herbie said, "That bitch can't cook a damn thing!"

I turned to Aggie. "Did you hear that? I wouldn't take that. I'm sure you cook just fine."

"Dat lil' mothafucka don't know shit!" she said of Herbie.

I then turn to Herbie and said, "I wouldn't let any woman talk to me that way!"

"Fuck you, you fat bitch!" he said.

Again, I turn back towards Aggie and basically push her over the edge by saying, "I can't believe it. Nobody would ever say that to me and get away with it!"

Well that was it. She started after him and hit him right in the mouth and knocked him right on his ass. Herbie was either numb with alcohol or just didn't see it coming, because a blind man could have seen this punch coming down the pike. He angrily looked up at her and kicked at her two or three times just to keep her off of him. With the third kick, he hit one of her knees, causing her massive bulk to buckle.

As she started to lose her balance she grabbed at a chair, but she's too big for the chair to help her regain her stability and over she went along with the chair. She is now so mad and screaming at Herbie so hard that neither Dave nor I can understand what she is saying. Whatever it was, it wasn't pleasant. She looked like a giant sea turtle on its back trying in vain to right itself. The big chair lying on top of her was not helping matters either. At this time Dave was more than a little nervous.

"Man, we've got to call the police," he said reaching for our walkie-talkie.

"No, wait a minute," I said. "I told you, this is an event. You've got to see this. Like I said on the way over here, they've been going at it like this for years!"

After great effort, Aggie finally got to her feet and for a solid three minutes or more they cussed and screamed at the top of their lungs. Aggie made her way to Herbie and each of them were throwing anything within arms reach at each other. Through it all Dave and I were being richly entertained. I mean it's not everyday you see two grown people putting on a show like this.

As usual, Aggie got the upper hand and gave Herbie a four or five punch beat down. She snatched him off of the floor and threw him about five feet through the air, right into the wall next to the front door. As stereotypical as it may sound, a picture fell from the wall that Herbie just collided with; hitting him on top of his head. I couldn't believe it. Aggie then grabbed a large porcelain lamp with a heavy plaster base and was going to hit Herbie with it.

Well, Dave and I couldn't allow that or Herbie would have quite possibly had been the one who needed the ambulance. I grabbed hold of Aggie and the lamp she was carrying and slowed them both down a little bit. Being less than half the size of Aggie, I knew that I couldn't hope to stop her, so I delayed her arrival to Herbie's side by getting in her way and pushing her back. My delaying tactic gave Dave enough time to get Herbie to his feet and get him hustled through the front door and out into the yard.

Once Herbie was safely in the front yard, Dave finally called the city police for assistance. We couldn't leave them alone and I sure as heck didn't want to take either of them to the hospital. But, Aggie wasn't done. When she saw Herbie standing in the front yard she started hurling insults and anything at him that she could get her hands around. Their yard was littered with all kinds of stuff including cans, bottles, magazines, shoes, silverware, and a footstool.

After the "event" spilled into the front yard, it only took the police a minute to arrive and restore the peace. If the cops would have known how this all happened in the first place, I would have had some explaining to do. On the other hand, some good did come from this latest episode and misadventure of unrequited love. Aggie forgot all about needing that ambulance.

Chapter 13
JESUS...AND THE MIRACLE OF PRAYER

Once in a great while, there comes along an ambulance call that is truly remarkable or so unusual, that it is reminisced in EMS circles for years and years. Such is the "Jesus" call—or more aptly put, the "JEEE-SUUS" call. Several years ago on a hot and sunny summer Sunday afternoon, our dispatch center received a call for the urgent need of an ambulance at a local neighborhood church. My partner at the time was a guy by the name of Bill Boyd. We had grown up together and were members of the same high school graduating class. We had many of the same friends, classes, and interests, and now we both were paramedics.

On this particular day, Bill and I are sitting at the central station just passing the time by watching TV, reading the local newspapers, or just conversing with our in-house dispatcher. It was kind of a lazy afternoon and Bill and I hadn't done much all morning. At about 4 p.m. the emergency lines were starting to ring in the dispatch office. Before we knew it, most of the company was busy with various types of ambulance calls.

As we sat there we heard the call that neither of us would ever forget. We were able to listen in on the conversation between the caller and our dispatcher by listening to a speaker that was tapped into the emergency phone lines. This was done so as the duty crews would have a "heads-up" on what kind or type of call was coming in. I remember thinking that this particular caller sounded like he was describing a cardiac arrest.

Up until this time, it had been a lazy day. I was in no mood to run a cardiac arrest call. However, the business of EMS is pretty much an "anything, anytime" kind of a business. So with the thought of my peaceful and tranquil day swiftly coming to an end, we quickly got underway and blazed over to the local church.

When we arrived, we saw about three dozen people waving their arms as to flag us down. Once we pulled into the parking lot area, there were still others pointing, shouting, and yelling. I thought, *with the number of people outside the church working to get Bill and me into the church, was anybody helping the poor soul who was in need of our assistance in the first place?*

As we came to a stop, there were several people who waded up to, and crowded around the ambulance. Some of them were offering to help us carry in some of the many pieces of equipment that we needed. Others were imploring us to hurry up and get into the church. Still others were trying to tell us what had happened.

As I have no less than a dozen people telling me these things (all at the same time), I cautiously jumped out of the front passenger seat and just yelled out to the crowd, "Does anybody know for sure whether or not the patient is breathing?"

It wasn't unanimous, but most of the people thought that the elderly gentleman was not breathing. So, of the people who offered to help, I loaded the impromptu volunteers with our cardiac monitor, airway box, portable suction unit, IV/drug box, and an oxygen bottle. Two other men helped by removing and carrying the ambulance cot. I grabbed the blood pressure cuff and my personal stethoscope and all of us hustled up the several steep steps that led us into the church.

As we entered the main area of the church, there may have been 200 or more people in attendance. We saw about eight to ten people huddled over someone lying supine on the floor in front of the pulpit. It was obvious that nobody was doing CPR or for that matter, any kind of resuscitation. What was clear was that the only thing happening there was a prayer vigil.

Once Bill and I arrived at the patient's side, we saw this little, old, and very frail African-American man lying on his back. It was obvious from the pupils of his partially-closed eyes being fixed and dilated, along with the mucous membranes around his eyes (being very pale and no apparent signs of breathing), that he was indeed dead. My personal thoughts aside, my medical evaluation and many years of experience told me this wasn't going to end well.

When we quickly came to the patient's side, the pastor of the church was the only one of the prayer vigil who didn't scatter once we neared the patient's flank. As I knelt at the head of the patient, I looked up at the pastor who was standing next to me just pouring sweat out and asked him if he knew if anyone had attempted to do CPR.

He looked at me with a slight grimace and said, "Oh no, no. We didn't do anything like that. No."

Bill and I made brief eye contact to confirm to each other what we had just heard, and what it meant for the rapidly dwindling chances for a successful resuscitation effort. Bill immediately started chest compressions, and I opened our airway box as to retrieve the Ambu-bag and intubation equipment. After giving a few breaths to our patent with the bag, I quickly placed an endotracheal tube into his trachea to secure his airway, and then started breathing for him. Once we knew for sure that we were to be working a cardiac arrest, and since there were no MFR's dispatched or able to respond to this emergency, we called for a secondary ambulance for assistance.

At the time, our dispatcher informed us that Medic was still getting hammered with calls for paramedics to respond to the scene of a child struck by a car while riding a bicycle, and to the home of someone with chest pain. There was also a baby delivery call on hold until one of our ambulances' could respond from a distant satellite station. What it meant to us, was that the other ambulances were either busy or way out of position, and therefore would be unable to come to our assistance in a timely fashion.

So, Bill and I would be the only EMS personnel to come to the aid of this victim of cardiac arrest and in all likelihood, make a vain attempt to save his life. As soon as I had our patient intubated and placed him on oxygen, I took over the CPR from Bill and did both the chest compressions and the ventilations. That freed up Bill to look for and to secure an IV site. Once my partner had secured the IV, and made a willing parishioner an IV pole, he placed our patient on the cardiac monitor and immediately started drug therapy.

During this whole time, there was no shortage of emotion. Some were complaining that we weren't doing things fast enough. Others were yelling for us to get the patient to the hospital. Several were just yelling at the thought of someone collapsing and dying in front of them. A precious few people were inquiring whether they could do something to help us with our rescue efforts. Usually that's a good thing, but other than the gentleman who was holding the IV for us— and since it takes a lot of training to help and not to be just in the way— there wasn't much the congregation could do "physically."

One of the things that I noticed when Bill and I entered the church was that about five or six feet behind the pulpit was a chorus. The chorus was ten people in length and three people in depth. Of the ten columns across, each column had a microphone secured on a stand, and a loud speaker in front of each of the microphones. At the time I didn't think much of it. The ladies who were members of the chorus were just standing there and watching the events unfold five feet in front of them.

I've come to realize that when people don't know what to do, they'll usually do something, even if it's counterproductive. During the early minutes of the resuscitation efforts, and amidst the yelling and some complaining, we started to hear a rhythmic sound from our large audience. It was sort of soft at first. Then it became louder and still louder. I couldn't understand it at first, but what Bill and I were listening to, was that a few members of the congregation in their attempts to do "something" to help. They were chanting, "Jesus.... Jesus.... Jesus.... Jesus."

In a matter of just a few short minutes, more and more people were joining in and chanting, "Jesus, Jesus." Except now it was more like "Jeee-suus.... Jeee-suus.... Jeee-suus,...." That spread like wild fire and suddenly the thirty-member chorus, with their loud speakers on, and most likely the vast majority of the rest of the congregation, were chanting in the same loud, rhythmic tone, "Jeee-suus, Jeee-suus," However, it was now like, "JEEE-SUUS, JEEE-SUUS, JEEE-SUUS, JEEE-SUUS," as the organist joined in.

It became so incredibly loud that I could feel the floor shaking. I distinctly remember looking up over my head, just to see if anything other than possibly the roof that might at any moment fall in on us. Luckily for us, nothing would be falling our way. As Bill and I are continuing our efforts in what would eventually be a fruitless attempt to save this little old man's life, it became increasingly more difficult for Bill and me to communicate with each other over the pounding noise.

In most cases, two paramedics with the years of experience that Bill and I had, could run a call with nothing much needed to be said between us. However, due to the intricacies and safety concerns that are inherent in treating a cardiac arrest, you need to talk or at least communicate by making gestures or signaling.

During the course of treatment, the man's heart rhythm changed from a flat line (or what we call asystole) to a fibrillation. That meant it was time to defibrillate our patient in an attempt to "jump-start" his heart. We couldn't hear a sound from each other and as a result, when Bill placed the defibrillation paddles on the man's chest to deliver the shock, he looked right at me and mouthed the word "clear." As I raised my hands from off the man's chest as well as dropping the bag that we used to ventilate him with, Bill quickly pressed the red discharge buttons on the defibrillator paddles and delivered the required electrical shock.

When that amount of energy is delivered there is a body wide muscle contraction. The phenomenon that happens more times than not is that the moment the electricity hits and charges through the body, the arms, legs, and even the patient's head and neck contract. On occasion, it even appears the patient bends a little bit at the waist. This is particularly true of smaller, skinnier people. And as I said, he was a tiny, little, frail man.

During this particular cardiac arrest, I remember the man's body contractions appeared very violent. So when Bill pressed the buttons on the defibrillator, and as I was raising my hands from the patient, it appeared that somehow the patient was raising his arms toward my hands. Later I was told that it looked like "I" was raising, or attempting to raise this dead man. I didn't know it at the time, but as Bill defibrillated the patient perhaps at least a half dozen times over the first twenty minutes, people were having a tough time watching what we were doing.

I guess it explains the screaming, yelling, and the crescendo in the chanting that happened every single time the patient was defibrillated. The whole episode was a heartbeat from pure pandemonium. At this point, whenever we defibrillated our patient it broke some of the people out into frenzy. I glanced toward the congregation and saw several people sitting, leaning, slumped over, lying on the pews, and looking like they were all on the verge of passing out.

Some of the well-intentioned ladies were standing in a small huddle a few feet from our side, weeping uncontrollably. Others were busy fanning those who appeared to be in distress, all the while still chanting "JEEE-SUUS.....JEEE-SUUS....JEEE-SUUS....."

Bill wasn't helping matters either. Somehow, both of us were finding it strangely humorous that whenever we had to defibrillate our patient, that we knew people in the crowd around us would be just coming unglued. After about the third or fourth defibrillation, we couldn't even look at each other for the fear of laughing out loud. God knows that not a soul in the place would have, or could have heard us laugh, but it would have been plain as day to see, and that would not have been good.

Here we are, just doing the best that we can, and coming up just short of biting a hole in each of our respective lips to keep from laughing our heads off. Don't misunderstand, whether we laughed or not doesn't mean that there would have been a difference in our care or the treatment that we rendered; it just would have looked extremely unprofessional. It would have been in incredibly bad taste. But, I would also be less than honest if I didn't say that it was all that I could do as to keep a straight face.

As it turned out, I don't think anyone even noticed our struggle with maintaining our proper composure. We continued our physically demanding CPR efforts, and the majority of the congregation continued their efforts as well. Soon everyone had joined hands and the pastor of the church was at the head of the line with his hands on my shoulder. I could only assume it was to channel or transmit divine power our way to assist in the life-saving efforts. By this time my ears were ringing and my head was spinning from the noise and commotion of the event.

After nearly thirty minutes, we finally got another crew to assist us. Both Ray Horton and Chris Forbaugh were a welcomed relief. What Ray and Chris saw when they arrived at our side, due to the heat of the summer day, was the result of the intense physical work Bill and I were performing. We were two sweat-soaked and physically spent paramedics.

As our colleagues joined in, Ray kneeled down next to me to take over chest compressions.

He yelled directly into my ear, "What is going on here?" Noticing the shaking floor he said, "Is this place coming apart or what?"

"Good God, I hope not! It's been like this for at least twenty minutes!" I said.

Ray started chest compressions while Chris helped Bill with the needed IV drug therapy and patient assessment. I continued breathing for the patient by ventilating him with our bag resuscitator. Even with the four of us, it was still so loud that we didn't have much better luck in communicating with one another than just the two of us had. Through it all, we continued our efforts until we knew we had exhausted every opportunity the patient presented to us.

Finally, the decision was made to remove our patient from the church and transport him to the local hospital. Chris retrieved a backboard from our ambulance. He came back into the church with it and while we were still doing CPR, we placed the patient on top of the backboard so we could lift him onto the ambulance cot. It also provided us with a stiff surface in which to continue our vigorous CPR.

Once we started to wheel the patient out of the church, many members of the congregation followed us to the doors. At that time, most of them had quieted down considerably, the organist had stopped playing, and the choir stopped chanting. Several gentlemen helped us carry the cot with our patient on it down the eight or ten steps to the ground level, and then out to the parking lot to where our ambulance was parked.

Others helped us by carrying the many pieces of equipment from out of the church. As we loaded our patient into the back of the ambulance, I made it a point to thank everyone who helped with our efforts, and especially those who helped carry the many items as well as the cot back out to our ambulance.

The pastor also followed us as we exited the church, but then turned and walked quickly toward his car and proceeded to drive to the local hospital where we were taking our patient. Once we loaded the patient into the back of the ambulance, I climbed in with him and quickly resumed CPR. One of the guys who arrived to back us up, asked whether I wanted or needed any help with CPR, or help in continuing any of the advanced life support measures that we had been performing. I told both Ray and Chris that I thought that we were pretty much finished doing any drug therapy, and that I would just be doing CPR during our expedited five to six minute trip to the hospital. At the time, we believed that it would be in everyone's best interest if Ray and Chris remained available to respond to another emergency call if necessary.

The trip to the hospital was uneventful as far as anything changing in our patient's condition. As we arrived at the emergency room, the pastor of the church was already waiting for us at the ambulance entry point. As my partner pulled the ambulance to a stop, I could see him walking very briskly toward us. Bill left the driver's seat and quickly opened the doors in the back of the ambulance. I momentarily stopped doing chest compressions just long enough to jump out and help get the cot out. I then restarted the CPR and the pastor enquired as how his parishioner was coming along. I told him that it didn't look good as we rolled the cot past him and into emergency room.

The truth of the matter was that from the very minute that Bill and I arrived at the church, both of us understood that if this feeble old man would ever survive the ordeal it would be a miracle. Another truth is, that since we as paramedics treat cardiac arrest victims the same exact way that in-hospital doctors and nurses do, the chances of a victim of cardiac arrest responding differently to the hospital staff is about zero.

Our patient was transferred from our cot to an emergency room bed, Bill consulted with the attending physician and nurses on what had transpired, and what course of treatment was given. I had a chance to visit and talk with the pastor. He was still shook-up over the whole event, and said that he had never been as surprised, and shocked when our patient collapsed right in front of him at the church. The pastor was still wiping the perspiration off of his forehead, just as he was during our time at the church.

He then said to me, "I want to thank you. You boys did just great! And we did all we could do, too. You know we were really working hard for that man! I guess after all of that, if the Lord wants you, I guess you're going with Him and that's that."

I responded with my head still buzzing and echoing with the noise of the well-intended members of his congregation. I gave him a smile and a handshake and agreed.

"The people in your congregation were all working really hard. Heck, even your organist was doing what she could do. I want you to know that Bill and I did appreciate everyone's good intentions. But you're right. I guess when it's your time, it's your time."

I also told him that the four of us who came to the aid of his parishioner did what we all thought was best and that we worked as hard as we could. I did tell him though that at the onset, I thought the man's chances for ultimate survival were bleak at best. The pastor was right about one thing; you just do all that you can do and you do it the best you can.

When I think of the intensity of the well-intentioned parishioners, the pastor, organist, choir, I think of the deafening noise. When I remember the look on Ray Horton's face when he and Chris Forbaugh arrived to assist Bill and me, I think of disbelief, bewilderment, and perhaps a little amusement. When I think of Bill defibrillating the patient who looked like I'm magically raising the dead—forgive me, I just have to laugh out loud.

***

I was working at our central station with a basic EMT by the name of Nate Hamilton. Nate is really a great guy who always endeavors to do the right thing. He always works hard and is a terrific support person for the paramedic who he is assigned to work with.

We were at our central station catching a quick bite to eat when our dispatcher informed us that there was a report of an elderly woman who was found not breathing. When our dispatcher inquired whether or not she had a pulse, the daughter who discovered her said that she didn't think so. With that information we jumped into our ambulance and sped to the address we were given. After being en route for only a minute or so, I contacted our dispatcher for an update on the condition of our patient and to inquire if someone was doing CPR. Our dispatcher said that she tried to give her daughter instructions over the phone on how to start CPR but the caller declined the information and said her mother was cold to the touch.

The woman stated that she would wait until EMS arrived to assess her mother. At that point I wondered aloud to Nate that the lady we were rushing to see must be really cold and really dead. And if that was indeed the case, why were we hustling to this address if our patient's own daughter isn't lifting a finger to help her. With no further information or consideration, I concluded that she must have been dead for several hours. With that thought, I shut our emergency lights off and drove the normal traffic speed to our destination.

Once we arrived and parked the ambulance at the apartment building, we were met there by a patrolman from the local city police department who arrived just moments earlier. It was their police department that received the initial 9-1-1 call so he responded to this emergency call moments before the police dispatcher notified our ambulance service.

As he exited his squad car and walked toward the ambulance he asked if we needed any help carrying equipment. I told him that it sounded like we had an elderly woman upstairs who in all likelihood had been dead for hours so there wasn't going to be much to do on this particular call. Nate retrieved the stretcher out of the back of the ambulance and I opened an outside compartment, grabbed a body bag, tossed it on the cot, and the three of us walked into the building.

Since local police protocol requires a written report on every dead body they encounter, the officer rode in the elevator with us. The woman's apartment, was a few short steps down a narrow hallway. We entered the living room area where we were introduced to our patient's daughter and husband, and an elderly woman who was sitting in a wheelchair. As I looked at the woman in the wheelchair, she was slumped heavily to her left side with her left arm hanging down with her fingertips nearly touching the carpeted floor. From a glance of five feet away the patient was absolutely still.

At that moment I turned my attention to the daughter and inquired as to what happened. She said she had last talked with her mother at about 7 a.m., and she seemed just fine. Her mother hadn't complained about any particular pain, discomfort or trouble breathing. After her early morning call, she had attempted to reach her by phone several more times after first talking with her but was unsuccessful. By mid-evening she became concerned about not reaching her mother and decided to go across town to investigate. She then said that she found her mother ten minutes ago, just as she presented to us now.

Not expecting much at all, I walked around to the front of her wheelchair and looked at her chest to see whether she was breathing or moving any air at all. Not seeing the slightest movement, I knelt in front of the lady. She looked pale, gray and slightly cyanotic. Her eyes were half open, pupils non-reactive, and she had that thousand-yard stare that says, "Dead, gone, and not coming back."

I reached for her dangling arm to feel for a radial pulse and was not at all surprised that she was as cold as ice and without a pulse. I got up off of my knee, stepped to the back of the wheelchair, placed my hands on either side of her neck, and straightened her head in a last attempt to find any clinical signs of life. I had my latex-gloved hands on her cold neck, and my eight fingers were in a search for a carotid pulse.

I felt for perhaps twenty seconds and felt nothing. I gently laid her head back to the left side, turned to her daughter, and told her that she was right, her mother was gone. I extended my condolences to the family and friends present, and told the police officer that when he finished getting all of the pertinent information on the dead woman's name, age, date of birth, etc., that I would need a copy of it.

Nate asked me at that time if I wanted him to go down to the ambulance and get the cardiac monitor in order to run a cardiac strip and confirm her death. I told him that since her dangling arm was as cold as could be and already slightly stiff, that the monitor wouldn't be necessary.

I told her daughter that protocol dictated that I call the hospital and advise the emergency department that we had a body, and inform the staff of the circumstances of the death. After that I would have to call the on-call medical examiner, her doctor, and (if the dead woman's doctor is agreeable to sign the death certificate) a funeral home. If the doctor is not willing or able to sign the death certificate, we would have to bag her and take her to the hospital's morgue. Along with the usual paperwork, it's quite the process and can take well over an hour to complete.

I asked the daughter where her mother kept her phone. She motioned to me that it was right around the corner in her kitchenette. I called the emergency department using the usual phone number reserved for EMS providers so we could either talk directly to a doctor or more often than not an RN. After hearing the phone ring two or three times, one of the emergency department's registered nurse's, Erin, answered the phone.

Due to the close proximity of the immediate family and a few friends who arrived shortly after we were summoned, I greeted Erin with a serious and professional demeanor. I began to tell her of the call that we were on, and that we had a body we needed to take care of. I got as far as telling Erin that the woman had not been seen in perhaps as long as twelve hours, when I heard several of the people just eight feet from me talking in unison.

During my time on the phone, the daughter's husband (who was a local minister) and several deacons of the church, along with the daughter, started to pray. I didn't think much about it. At the scene of ambulance calls it's not unusual for me to hear people pray for help and healing of someone gravely ill or injured, or for the soul and peace for those who are gone.

I wasn't listening to what the specific words of the prayer were, but I knew that was what the family was doing. As the prayer continued, I was talking to Erin about our dead patient, and giving her all of the particulars.

About a minute into my conversation, suddenly, loudly, and out of the blue, my partner yelled, "Jim, she just took a breath!"

My first reaction was, did I just hear what I thought I heard? A second later when Nate's statement sunk in, my next reaction was of irritation. I was sure that the loud and unabashed statement made by Nate was going to get the family and friends all in an uproar over something that was not there. Now I'm going to have to go back into the living room and be the bad guy, and reiterate my findings to the family, and dash any hopes they may have for the lady's survival. At the same time I'm wondering if my partner is, or should be on the list for a brain transplant.

I told Erin that I now didn't know for sure what was going on and that I would give her a call back in a few minutes. I hung up the phone and was ready to chastise my partner for being an idiot. I must have looked irritated when I came from behind the small wall that divided the living room area from the kitchenette because Nate took a step or two backward, and looked rattled and a little intimidated.

He quickly recovered and said, "Jim, I'm telling you, she just took a breath!"

"Nate, how can that be? I checked her thoroughly. She doesn't have a pulse. Her eyes are fixed, she's not breathing and she is as cold as ice! On top of that, her arm is getting stiff."

At that particular moment, her daughter stepped forward and said in a matter of fact tone, "I know she has a bad arm!"

Wide-eyed and excited Nate pipes up again, "I don't know what to tell you, but she just took a breath. I saw her take one!"

At that moment the prayer session abruptly stopped and the daughter was now realizing what might be happening. She had the biggest shocked look on her face and blurted out, "Can that be? Can she still be alive?"

With the thought of there not being the smallest chance possible, I said, "Well, we can take a look again."

Once again I knelt down beside the patient as I did before, and looked at her just in time to see her take the shallowest of breaths. I must have done a double take because Nate said in an excited tone, "See, I told you! She just took another breath!"

"Jesus, you're right!"

I scrambled to my feet. I tilted her head to a mid-line position and felt for a pulse. What I felt was as shocking as it was unbelievable. She not only had a pulse that I or any EMS provider might at best expect to be thready and irregular (if she had one at all), but she had a pulse that was as regular as clockwork and as strong as could be. It was so strong I felt sure that I could have felt it through a baseball player's glove. There was definitely no problem with detecting a pulse where just a short two minutes ago, unquestionably no pulse existed. To say I couldn't believe it would be the understatement of the century! I was absolutely astounded!

Without assessing her breathing I yelled to Nate, "Get her on the floor! Help me get her on the floor!"

Nate snapped into action and together we quickly lifted her out of her wheelchair and got her laying flat on the floor in a supine position. Although she may have started to breath adequately, I didn't wait to see. I quickly opened her airway by raising her neck and tilting her head back. Within five or ten seconds she started taking deep, lung-filling breaths.

Nate quickly got our cot from the hallway just outside our patient's apartment, and the police officer helped him get it next to where our patient was laying. Within the last ninety seconds I felt like I was in the

"Twilight Zone." I wasn't at all sure I wasn't asleep somewhere and just dreaming about this event. I felt that at any time I would awaken in my own bed, scratching my head over a really odd dream. I say that because at that precise moment, I wasn't sure what was real and tangible and what was fictitious and surreal. As a longtime EMS provider and a man of biosciences that's a very uncomfortable feeling and a bad position to be in.

While the seconds rolled by and the ambulance cot was being wheeled into the apartment, I began to contemplate what I witnessed. And as difficult as it is to imagine, not knowing what to think or do, I just about began to cry. The family was also rejoicing with hugs and kisses, jumping up and down, and praising God for what they too had borne witness to. Nate and I quickly unfurled the cot blanket and sheet, promptly scooped her up, and laid her on our stretcher. We covered her, gave her oxygen by mask, and with her personal information and her prescription medicines in hand, we got her into the elevator, downstairs, and into our ambulance just as quickly as humanly possible.

Earlier, when we were asking the family members present about the medical history of our would be patient, we found out that she was a diabetic. With that information, we did a blood glucose level test on her and found that her blood glucose level was at 24mg. /dl of blood. That is very low, and would almost always render someone unconscious. However, it would not have anything to do with her having no pulse. Even if it had, I didn't do anything for her low blood sugar until after we got her into the ambulance.

Once we loaded her into the ambulance, we jumped into the patient compartment with her. Nate recorded her blood pressure, heart rate, and placed her on our cardiac monitor. While he was doing that, I was busy preparing to start an IV so I could give her sugar (dextrose) in order to attempt to wake her up. On the way to the hospital, our patient was still unconscious and only improved negligibly. Not being medically sure at all of anything that has to do with our patient, I told Nate not to waste any time getting to the hospital.

As I sat on the bench seat opposite of where the patient was laying, I still couldn't believe what had just transpired. I kept saying over and over to myself, "How can this be? How can this be? This kind of thing just doesn't happen in science-based western-style medicine." It's as simple as that.

Once we arrived at the hospital, and turned the care of our patient to the emergency room staff. I retreated to the EMS report writing room clearly shaken to my core. I sat there for a solid fifteen minutes and didn't as so much as take my pen out of my uniform shirt pocket. I sat there thinking, contemplating, and reflecting on the incredible events of the last thirty or so minutes. I was still so emotionally wrung out it would not have taken much to bring me to tears.

Without a clue on what to write on my patient care report, I decided to take a short walk to the room where our patient was being treated. When I walked in, I saw our patient's daughter standing next to her mother beaming with joy and happiness. As I approached the two of them, the daughter turned to me, extended her hand, and said, "Thank you so much."

"Don't thank me. I didn't do a meaningful thing until we got Mom into the back of the ambulance."

I saw the hospital staff had a heated blanket on her and remembering how cold she was in her apartment, I asked one of the nurses present what was her current temperature. She told me that she had just recorded a rectal temperature of 88.6 degrees Fahrenheit; that's a body core temperature more than a full ten degrees below what's considered normal. I could only imagine how cold her arms and legs must have been.

For me, there is no doubt that I experienced the most incredible event possible that, to this day gives me chills. With my eyes I witnessed the most spiritual and faith-based event in all of my years in EMS. In my mind, I experienced the most extraordinary gift possible that to this day is scientifically unexplained, and lends credence and credibility of the work of a higher power, and leaves me with a feeling of divinely inspired awe and gratitude.

Without reservation, I readily and honestly admit that this happening left me not only shaken to the core of my professional being, but also my mortal being as well. To this day, I truly believe what I witnessed was nothing short of the unfathomable power of a God-given miracle. I mean that with all of the feeling, sincerity, and gravitas that I can communicate on these pages.

For the record, when I finished talking to our patient's daughter—which was only three or four minutes—the lady I took for long dead and gone, was now fully conscious, alert, and oriented to her surroundings. Suddenly, she was able to hold her own and participate in a protracted conversation with her daughter as well as the nurses.

I extended my heartfelt well wishes to them both and left the room shaking my head at the emotionally charged amazement of this particular ambulance call. It was one of the rarest events I've ever witnessed in my long and winding EMS career.

Chapter 14
JUST ANOTHER DAY

The following is another day in the life of an ordinary EMS provider—me. This is what I did, who I saw, and how my partner and I impacted the people we were called to help. This is a fairly typical day of a twenty-four hour shift at our central station in Benton Harbor, Michigan.

Not all of the calls I ran on this particular shift originated in Benton Harbor, or even the large townships which surround it. It is however, what can, and is expected when one comes to work as a paramedic at Medic 1 Ambulance. Rod was my partner for the shift.

7:57 a.m. – As usual I flew into work and punched in about 7:57 a.m. I don't know why, but I always seem to barely get to work on time. Other guys show up anywhere from fifteen to forty-five minutes before their scheduled time to be on-duty. Somehow I just have to hit that snooze alarm just one more time. My only saving grace is that I almost always have my uniform ready to throw on, or it's hanging on a hook in my car.

At the station there is the usual hustle and bustle of about fifteen people all milling around the common kitchen and television area. Not only are they EMS road personnel, but also office, supervisory and members of our wheel-chair division. Most everyone coming into work is relatively pleasant; except for the two cranky ambulance crews just getting off a twenty-four hour shift. I come with my duffle bag with all kinds of personal items in it, including clothing, food and drink for the day, a magazine or two, a flashlight and my own stethoscope.

After a little small talk with my colleagues I inquire the where-abouts of Rod. There is word that he is checking out the ambulance making sure we have all the state-mandated items needed for our shift. He also checks for all of that, plus all of the mechanical things, such as the running lights, emergency lights, various engine fluids, siren, emergency radios, etc. He even has it down to where he supplies the type and size of latex gloves that I like to use.

I go to help him but he is already done. We head back into the living areas of the station to complete station duties that may include making up your bed for the day, sweeping the carpeted floors, cleaning up the kitchen area, etc. It doesn't take more than twenty minutes.

9:14 a.m. (Call #1) - "You have a P.I. (personal injury) accident at Lemon Creek and Hollywood Roads. A man is reported lying in the street. Handle priority 1."

That's all we know and that's all we have to go on until the police or a Medical First Responder gets on scene to update us on the condition of our soon to be patient. As I climb into the ambulance and fasten my seat belt, Rod gets behind the steering wheel, fastens himself in, flips the emergency lights and siren on and we're off and running. It just so happens that this particular call is a long way out of our normal service area, so it takes us about eight minutes to reach our destination.

As we rolled up to the call, it's in a hilly part of the road. The police are there as are several bystanders. The good citizens have done their best to keep this patient warm by heaping blankets on top of him. It's in the first week of February, so there is snow and ice on the roads and it's plenty cold.

Rod gets the ambulance properly parked and I scrambled out and run to the side of our patient. He was awake and appeared to be alert and oriented. I asked what happened and this man (in his mid-30s) says that while he was driving on the ice and hard packed snow he lost control of his vehicle. He then informed me that he decided to jump out of his car before he hit a tree.

My first thought was, *okay, I'm not talking to the smartest guy I'm going to see today.* Then I considered my decades-long work in EMS and conclude that this guy just might be the smartest guy that I see today; who knows. To contemplate that possibility doesn't surprise me at all but it does make me cringe a little. At the present I'm really hoping that the latter thought won't be the case! As I look him over he tells me he has abdominal pain on his left side and his right forearm has pain.

Due to the mechanism of injury (in this case jumping/falling out of a car at an unknown speed) this man needs to have Central Nervous System (CNS) precautions taken. Already Rod has the appropriate cervical collar and a backboard out of the ambulance. By the time I get done with a rough assessment, Rod is ready to get our patient on to the spine board and get him out of the snow and cold. I'm ready too.

We fit the man with a collar to keep his neck immobile and then roll him gently with the aid of two police officers and a bystander onto the backboard. A minute later we have him secured firmly and loaded into the ambulance. Shortly thereafter and after a more extensive secondary examination, including assessing vital signs, lung sounds and a basic neurological check, I concluded that our patient most likely didn't have any internal injuries and that advanced life support (ALS) would not be necessary.

We were on the scene of the accident a total of nine minutes and we arrived at the hospital exactly forty minutes from when we first received the call for help. After ambulance cleanup, restock and the ever-present paperwork, we left the hospital at about 10:30 a.m. We found out later, our patient was later discharged with superficial injuries.

10:50 a.m. (Call #2) - We were called to a local hamburger joint for a woman experiencing chest pain. The woman was a worker there, but as Rod and I arrived we found her sitting in one of the booths awaiting our arrival. My first impression was that she really wasn't in much distress at all. She had no facial grimaces and her eyes as well as the tone of her voice didn't tell us that her pain was at this moment present, let alone significant. She spoke in long sentences rather than short, pain interrupted phrases. So after talking with her for no more than thirty seconds, I'm skeptical about this so-called emergency.

She told us that she was in her early 30s and had been working in the kitchen area when she suddenly experienced sharp, shooting chest pain and that it hurt worse when she took in a deep breath. She said that she called us immediately after she had the very first pain. I was beginning to think we're dealing with either a hypochondriac or someone who doesn't want to work today. Her vital signs were great. Her lungs sounds were clear and dry.

She was alert and oriented. She had no medical history concerning heart or cardiovascular issues. Lastly, and perhaps most importantly, she wasn't taking nor had she taken any medication that would indicate any kind of heart or cardiovascular problem.

After spending less than ten minutes examining her, we advised she probably in all likelihood didn't have a heart problem and to see her own physician if signs or symptoms persisted. We then called our medical control, which is the emergency room at the local hospital, to advise them of our patient, her complaint, our subsequent examination, and finally our no transport decision. The physician agreed with our overall assessment as well as our medical advice. We then cleared the call at 11:03 a.m.

Now at last, I had a little time to go back to the station and make myself a small breakfast. With EMS you never know when your next break will come so you take one whenever you can get it. Rod and I got over an hour break before our next call. We used that time to eat a couple of deluxe hamburgers that the manager of the restaurant gave us in appreciation of our caring attitude and professional demeanor.

12:14 p.m. (Call #3) -The next call was to a dental office located about a half mile from the resent chest pain complaint. I hadn't been to very many calls at dental offices but when I have, it's usually because some patient has had an adverse reaction to the local anesthetic that was being used, there's an anxiety attack in progress, or somebody has passed out. This time it was for neck pain.

As I start to think out loud I said to Rod, "Neck pain at the dentist's office? What's up with that?"

Unfortunately we were again several miles away sitting at our central station when the dispatch for help occurred. Once there we found a lady in her 40s lying supine on a hard-carpeted floor with a man holding her head. I guess he was doing this so she wouldn't attempt to move until we arrived. My thought was that someone tripped or stumbled and ended up with a minor ground-level fall.

Generally speaking, we don't do much with those types of calls unless there is a neurological deficit. I don't remember the last time someone was truly hurt falling onto a carpeted floor from a standing position that didn't at the least hit their head on something on the way down.

After a little inquiry, we found that the man holding her head was the dentist and the lady on the floor was his secretary. She was fully alert and oriented and then proceeded to tell me that while she was sitting at her desk she had a spontaneous and sudden onset of a very sharp pain sensation in her neck that made her nauseous. She also said that she "tingled all over" and she felt "empty inside" and that she very nearly passed out. I asked her if this had ever happened to her before. She said no, but that she had fractured her first cervical vertebrae in her neck about eighteen months ago.

After hearing the story of her neck fracture I thought to myself that this dentist isn't the putz that I first thought that he might be for holding her cervical spine in place. In all likelihood he knew of her medical condition and therefore just how serious this situation could be. An injury to the spinal column is never anything to take lightly. You never know whether there is a residual effect from the healing process that might be a problem, or whether there is now a related problem with scar tissue, or if the bone was perhaps not properly set or fused or the joint had deteriorated.

The one thing that I know, is that with a fracture that high in the neck, it is often deadly or conceivably worse. Our lady could become just a head on a pillow, if we don't handle her problem just exactly right. So with the good doctor's help, Rod and I fitted her carefully with a stiff-neck type of cervical collar, and very carefully secured her onto our backboard. We used towel rolls along either side of her neck, and duct taped her head and neck in place to the spine board.

We loaded her into the ambulance, started a normal saline IV, and took her to the nearest hospital which was only five miles away. Rod drove us over to the hospital and we arrived at 12:43 p.m. By the time we consulted with the nursing and medical staff in the emergency room, and finished our paperwork, it was 12:56 p.m. She had a CT scan that revealed no other injury, and was discharged from the emergency room with a prescription for a narcotic pain reliever.

Approximately one week after this particular event, she had sudden numbness in her right arm. This time she called her neurosurgeon and he immediately ordered her to have an MRI scan. That medical test showed a herniated disc between her fourth and fifth cervical vertebrae. Shortly thereafter, she underwent a surgical procedure to stabilize her neck and was back to work within six weeks.

12:57 p.m. (Call #4) -The phone rings in the EMS room at the local hospital. The EMS room is a small room just outside the emergency department that the hospital provides to the EMT's and paramedics to do our paperwork. It's also a place to keep our non-narcotic drug supplies as well as other equipment that may be left behind or attached to patients after we complete a call. I answered the phone and one of our dispatchers informs me that there is a lady in the emergency room who needs to be returned to her home. The dispatcher asks me that since we are there, would we be so kind as to take her back to her house?

The elderly lady was in her mid-70s and was not likely to see her next birthday. She has been stricken with colon cancer that has advanced to the stage where modern medicine can no longer do anything more to cure her or even at the least, prolong her life. Consequently, she is now under the palliative care of Hospice at Home. Hospice is a great organization that takes over the care and comfort for those who are at the end stages of life with terminal diseases and end of life medical disabilities.

By the time everything is in order with our next patient, it's almost a half hour before we're en route to her home. It only takes us five minutes to get her back to her house, but now since there is close to two feet of snow on the ground we have to wait to unload her from our ambulance because there is a medical equipment truck in the driveway. A family member came out of the house shortly after we arrived and asked if we could wait a couple of minutes. Apparently they had procured a hospital bed for their mother. After the man was done setting up her bed, he quickly got into his truck, and moved out of our way.

After getting our patient to her home, we found that getting her into the house, while on our ambulance cot, was going to present a couple of problems. First, there was no wheelchair ramp that led to any outside door and the four to five porch steps leading to her front door were icy, snow covered, and steep. Secondly, had we been able to get her to the front door, due to the size of our ambulance cot and the narrow entry points and sharp corner leading to her living room, we couldn't get her much past the front door.

So, with the help of a couple of stout family members we were able to get under the corners of the flat sheet she was laying on and kind of "hammock" her into the house and right onto her new bed. After we made her comfortable, I thanked her sons who had assisted us and wished them well with the care of their mother. I was relatively certain that they were going to have a tough time during the next few days or weeks.

No matter who you are, facing an expected end of life of a loved one is still a pretty tough thing to do. One of her sons then told me that the doctor had informed the family that their mother was now "actively passing away."

Rod and I finished and cleared from that call at 1:52 p.m.

A few hours later, the family called her doctor and before you could say, "Well that was a wasted trip," our other central ambulance was bringing her back for admission to the oncology floor at the very hospital in which Rod and I brought her from earlier in the day.

1:55 p.m. (Call #5)-Three minutes after getting our lady back to her home and into her hospital bed we received a call at an upscale nursing facility for a woman in her late 60s convalescing following a surgical repair for a broken hip. It seemed as though she had experienced some very uncomfortable, sharp chest pain. It took us nine minutes to arrive and in that period of time, the lady had informed us that upon our arrival, her chest pain was now completely gone.

Her husband had been notified before we were summoned and was at her bedside when we walked into her room. She was fairly indifferent of whether she wanted, needed or should go to the hospital. Of course after hearing the usual doom and gloom mantra that most ding-a-ling nurses give to some patients', the husband was all but insistent that we take her to the hospital. I told her husband that us taking her to the hospital would not be any problem at all, but we were going to check her out and give her an assessment before we would be taking her anywhere.

She was completely pain free and in no acute distress whatsoever. Her lungs were clear, full and dry and her vital signs were excellent and her skin was warm, pink, and dry. Rod hooked her up to our cardiac monitor and that also was showing a normal sinus rhythm. It's my policy that if I feel strongly enough about a patient's condition to warrant placing them on a cardiac monitor, then I will also start an IV on them as well. After that was done, we took another casual ride back to the hospital. It should be noted that after fully assessing her and discussing her condition with her and her husband and then having to listen to the nurse blather on and on, it took us twenty-seven minutes to get en route to the hospital.

Ten minutes later we arrived at the hospital with our pain-free patient with chest pain. Twelve minutes later, I was done with paperwork and Rod had gotten the ambulance restocked and back in order. As expected, she was checked over and sent back to the nursing home to continue her convalescence a short time later.

(Call #6) - Exactly one minute later, Rod and I were sent to see a female patient complaining about cramps to her arms and legs. We arrived to find a 39-year-old woman with a medical history of hypertension, insulin dependent diabetes (type 1), asthma, and arthritis. With that history she obviously had a problem with autoimmune diseases. God knows that all of that is a lot to live with, but she wasn't suffering directly or indirectly from any of those maladies. Her big complaint was simple cramps to her arms and legs that upon our arrival didn't seem to be serious or particularly painful. Even so, having a leg cramp in my opinion, it's never a reason to call for an ambulance.

After assessing and then walking our patient to the ambulance we got moving to the hospital. We called and advised the hospital staff of our assessment of the patient and what they could be expecting within the next five minutes. They summarily told us to admit her to the triage department. Basically, that's putting her in the waiting room and having her take her turn for non-emergency care like everybody else that did the responsible thing by seeking or finding their own transportation to the hospital. At times that might mean waiting for hours and hours until you can see a doctor. Most of the time, that's just the way that it is.

It's one of those countless times that tax dollars are needlessly spent on the same care that can be found and delivered at a small fraction of the price of going to an emergency room for non-emergency problems by simply visiting a walk-in clinic or your neighborhood doctor's office. It's also what happens when the recipient of that care doesn't have to spend a single dollar of their own money for the ambulance trip or any of the care they receive at the hospital. Eleven minutes later, our patient is sitting in triage and at 3:35 p.m. we're done with paperwork and ready to go again.

3:38 (Call #7) - I only had to wait a mere three minutes from being mildly irritated and annoyed to being red-faced angry. We were heading to a 30-year-old woman who was thirty-one weeks pregnant with her fourth child. She was complaining of lower abdominal pain. When we arrived, we gave her the usual list of questions that are unique to women who are pregnant. When is the baby expected? Has it been a normal pregnancy? How many times have you been pregnant? How many babies do you have right now? What medicines are you currently taking? Who's your doctor? The questions are extensive and important.

During the many questions posed to her, she informs us that her second and third children were stillborn (both at thirty-one weeks) from a condition called abruptio-placenta (when the placenta pulls away from the wall of the uterus). If it's a complete abruption, it means certain death for the baby. If it's a partial abruption, there is a chance for survival for the baby. If the uterus is damaged and bleeding, it can be life threatening for mom as well.

So with her description of the type of pain she is experiencing, and with her stated medical history, we have at last a bona-fide emergency on our hands. Right at this time she doesn't have any vaginal bleeding that would indicate an intra-uterine hemorrhage, but that's not always readily apparent. To us, it doesn't matter. With her symptoms and her history we start moving in a hurried fashion. Rod retrieves the cot from the ambulance as I finish my assessment.

I found that although she was experiencing abdominal pain her vital signs were all stable and unremarkable. Rod put her on oxygen and I started a large bore IV on her just in the event she starts to show any signs of acute internal bleeding. We're on scene for exactly ten minutes and now its lights and siren to the obstetrical floor at the local hospital. We arrived and have her upstairs in the obstetrical unit at 4:05 p.m.

Actually, I'm not mad yet.

We were instructed by the excellent nursing staff on the OB floor to take the patient to an exam room. As we quickly wheeled her into the room, one of the nurses is right behind us. As we got ready to move our patient to one of the beds the nurse says right out of the blue, "so Donna, when was the last time you smoked any crack?"

You could have knocked me over with a feather. It just never occurred to me that this woman who was pregnant with her fourth child was doing crack cocaine.

Not to be outdone, Donna said in a matter of fact tone, "Oh, I've been clean for two months."

Well, Hallelujah isn't that just great! She's been smoking crack cocaine right up to the end of her second trimester—that's if you believe what she is now telling you. As a general rule, I never believe anything a drug addict tells me. Although I don't know, I'd bet dollars to donuts that she was still smoking crack right up to the present time.

Shortly after I turned the care of this patient to the OB nursing staff one of the nurses informed me that it was documented that this is exactly what killed her second and third children. Now, I'm as mad as hell and I don't mind telling her so. Later I found out she was clean from any illicit drugs and summarily discharged back to her home. False alarm...this time.

What a disgusting creature she is and a great argument for sterilization. I fail to understand or to comprehend why people like her are not in prison. I'm certainly no lawyer, but I would think that a case for manslaughter might hold some water. After a brief but caustic rant, I finished my paperwork and again we're ready to go. It's now 1630 hours and as it turns out, Rod and I have a few minutes to catch our breath. We've had non-stop calls for four solid hours. Our respite lasts a short forty-five minutes.

4:30 p.m. (Call #8) - We left the hospital after our last call and stopped at a local deli to get Rod a sub sandwich. I had brought food from home. No sooner did we get a chance to grab a quick bite and we were off again. This time it is to back another one of our ambulances from our north area of emergency service.

There was a report of two people trapped inside a house fire. Fortunately, when a citizen reports a house fire and claims there are people inside the burning structure it's usually not the case. More often than not the caller just doesn't know the whereabouts of their neighbors or occupants. Not today. The local county sheriff's department sent a deputy to the location of the fire in case there would be a security issue, crime scene, to direct traffic or to somehow assist the all-volunteer fire department. As he arrived, he found that the firefighters had not yet arrived. He also found that there were indeed two elderly and somewhat infirm people still inside this burning house. As I understand it, he had to forcefully remove the old couple from their home.

As the Medic 1 ambulance arrived from the north area along with the fire department, the deputy had already pulled the old man into the still snow-covered yard. Apparently, he was badly burned and was suffering from smoke inhalation as well. The Medic 1 ambulance that covers our north area rushed him to the nearest hospital, but unfortunately he died just three hours later. The wife of the old man was no spring chicken, but she made it into the yard with no ill effects from the fire.

In response to the life-threatening emergency at hand or in an attempt to be heroic or at the least just trying to do the right thing for the right reason, the county deputy who pulled the two people from their burning home had gotten just a little bit too much smoke himself. After I checked out the elderly woman and found her to be completely void of any effects from the fire, I was informed by one of the volunteer firefighters at the scene that we needed to take a look at the deputy who ran into this house.

He told me that he had noticed that he was still coughing more than twenty minutes after he had exited the house. After talking to the deputy briefly, he did seem to still be in some minor to moderate distress. When I inquired whether he had any specific pain, he said he was essentially pain free. Mostly he just said that he felt like his lungs were on fire. I walked him over to where our ambulance was parked and did a more thorough exam on him. Rod put him on oxygen right away and we proceeded to get the man stripped down from the waistline, up.

After carefully listening to his lung sounds, I told him his lung sounds were fine but smoke inhalation will cause lung problems later rather than sooner. Smoke residue and ash were absent from his nasal and oral cavities and he had no signs of any pulmonary burns. He told me that the only Rx medicines that he takes are for his chronic hypertension. He wasn't kidding around about that. His blood pressure was 164/130. I told him that his pressure was high enough to ring the bell and that he really should keep a sharp eye on it and have it checked at different times of the day, regularly for the next couple of weeks. Being a 36-year-old African-American with a stocky build, I told him that he was much too young to be debilitated from a heart attack or a stroke.

He still really wasn't all that crazy about going to the hospital. That was still the case, up until the Sheriff himself found out what had just transpired. Another county deputy who was at the house fire but arrived after the fact, opened one of the back doors to our rig and said, "Sheriff Bailey said to take him to the hospital to be checked out. No questions asked."

Well that was that. It was a good decision. Even though he wasn't directly hurt from the fire, he really needed his blood pressure looked into. Besides a half an hour after this whole episode, his heart was still banging away at more than 120 beats per minute and his respiratory rate was still more than twenty times a minute. His vital signs told Rod and me that for whatever reason, his body was still under stress.

As a result, Rod put him on the heart monitor for me and I started an IV. Rod stuck a light probe on the end of his finger to measure the oxygen content in his blood. The pulse-ox reading told us that he was at one hundred percent, which was great. After we increased the rate in which we were giving him oxygen, his respiratory distress subsided and his other vital signs started to recede into the normal ranges of good health.

We arrived at the small community hospital at 6:01 p.m. and I finished up my paperwork a few minutes later. By the time I finished, Sheriff Paul Bailey was at the emergency room to look into the condition of his deputy.

Thankfully, the truly courageous police officer was released a few hours later from the hospital without any lingering effects from his ordeal.

6:43 p.m. (Call #9) - After we whizzed back into our central area, there was another call awaiting our arrival. We were dispatched to see a twenty-two year old female complaining that her "stomach hurt after a forceful bowel movement." (As a note, this is the nature and the frustration of EMS. You will be called to resuscitate a victim of a cardiac arrest or to hold someone's guts together following a stabbing or shooting and the next call is somebody having cramps following a bowel movement.)

We arrived at her house to find her in moderate distress. As with any sexually-active female of child-baring age, I inquired whether it was at all possible that she might be pregnant. She told me that her last menstrual period was two months ago. I asked if she had ever missed a period? She said she hadn't ever been late in that regard. Furthermore, there apparently was no bleeding or any kind of vaginal discharge. Since she was able to walk to the ambulance, she did.

Once we got her into the patient compartment of the ambulance, she said that it was too painful for her to sit on the bench seat. Reluctantly, we unfolded the cot so she could lie down on her left side. In that position, she seemed reasonably comfortable. As Rod drove the ambulance to the local hospital, I called the emergency room and advised the nursing staff of what we were coming in with.
I told the nurse who answered the phone that our patient was now laying on our cot as she was unable to sit. With that being said, the nurse advised me to take our patient to the triage department. Again, I told her that it would be inappropriate for my patient to go to triage because she would be unable to sit on a chair at all, let alone most likely several hours. She advised me that there were no beds available for her and that she didn't have much of a choice in the matter.

After my usual and brief conversation with the hospital personnel, I told our patient that she would have to sit in the waiting room at the hospital's emergency department. Still on our way to the hospital, she implored to me that she needed to lie on a bed because she felt that she just couldn't sit on a chair. Nonetheless, we arrived and wheeled her into the hospital waiting room still on our cot.

I told the triage nurse (a different nurse than I had spoken to five minutes earlier) that I didn't think that she could sit. Her reply was that she was busy and that we should do the best we can with her.

Our patient heard the same thing and was very reluctant to remove herself from our cot. I told her that I was really sorry but she didn't have an option in the matter. Almost crying, she got up and did attempt to sit on one of the cushioned chairs. Immediately it was obvious that it was much too painful. I told the nurse that this was totally unacceptable and if she couldn't find her a bed, then I would.

Now, I'm as mad as hell about this growing fiasco and I just couldn't believe that there wasn't a single bed available. To my disgust and surprise, there indeed was not a single bed to be had in the whole entire emergency department. As I stormed through the whole department and made my way back to the triage department, the triage nurse had the patient lying on a hospital sheet on the floor. I couldn't believe it. Now I'm not only disgusted, but mightily irritated.

I said to the nurse, "You've got to be kidding me! What are you wizards going to do if I happen to bring somebody in that happens to be unconscious?" She just looked at me and shrugged her shoulders.

Since I usually know when to say when, I just spun around to the patient and told her, "You should feel lucky. According to half of the billboards in the county, you're in the top one percent of all hospitals in the nation!"

I then briskly walked out of the triage department and into the EMS room and finished up the paperwork. We exited the emergency department and left the hospital at 7:50 p.m.

Later I found out that she was indeed, not pregnant and whatever her ailment may have been, she was later discharged from the emergency room.

8:14 p.m. (Call #10) - We were requested to go to one of the many area nursing homes to see a 90-year-old female with the complaint of her bleeding above the right eye. Usually it's because for whatever reason one of the clients has fallen. Either they fall out of bed or they stumble and fall in their attempt to walk by themselves to the restroom or something of that sort. Everyone in EMS is cognizant of the fact that someone falling at a nursing home and injuring themselves is not exactly unique.

We took our usual casual drive to the nursing home, unloaded our cot and proceeded to the patient's room. There we found a nurse "dabbing" the brow of a woman who was sitting in a wheel chair who didn't appear to be in any distress at all.

"What do you have there?" I asked.

With a straight face the nurse turns from her patient and says to me, "She fell five or six days ago and she keeps picking at the scab. Now it's bleeding again."

I'd like to say that I was surprised by what she said, but sadly, I wasn't. Nonetheless I couldn't help myself and I said back to her, "You called us because she keeps picking at a five day old scab and now it's bleeding?"

Of course that irritated the nurse and she says, "Well the doctor wants her evaluated."

I immediately thought to myself, "Yeah, right! What a crock. This is just one of those idiot nurses, who doesn't want to deal with this lady, so she calls the patient's doctor and paints a picture of trials, tribulations and probably a near-death experience."

Nonetheless, Rod and I lifted her off from her wheel chair and placed her gently on our cot. We wrapped her up with our sheet and blanket, scooped up the lady's pertinent medical information at the nurse's station and with a whole lot more EMS frustration we were off to the hospital with the most ridiculous call of the day. When we arrived at the hospital and wheeled our patient through the emergency room doors, the nurse, who I had talked to on the phone, was standing there, just staring at us.

Without saying a word to her, she says to me, "You've got to be kidding me?"

"Hey, ask dingle-belle at the nursing home about it. She's the resident wizard who thought that a leaky scab needed to be seen by you guys."

The other nurses at the hospital were just a little more than dismayed at why we were bringing this particular patient in. As I was concluding our usual paperwork on this truly waste of time and money call, we were on our way to our next call.

*The patient was returned within two hours back to the nursing home.

9:22 p.m. (Call #11) - The next call was to see a thirty-four-year-old female who reportedly had vaginal bleeding. The caller's location was a long way away and it took us eighteen minutes to arrive. We found our lady who was of eastern European descent hard to understand mostly because of her limited knowledge of the English language and my total lack of understanding the Russian language.

We finally realized that she was complaining of a heavier than usual bleeding for her usual monthly period and she stated that she had two periods last month. She said that she didn't have any pain but was really concerned about what might be going on with her. I checked her vital signs and lung sounds and found nothing out of the ordinary. I then asked what she wanted us to do for her and she just basically said that she didn't know whom she should call and she wanted us to tell her what she should do.

Apparently her husband, who is native to the United States, was out of town on business and it was just her and her nine-year-old daughter at home. It was obvious that she didn't want to have to take her daughter to the hospital with her. Finally, she called a friend to stay with her daughter and another friend to take her to the local emergency room. All of this took a while to accomplish and we didn't clear from that call until 10:10 p.m.

More than three and half hours later, our lady and her friend were quietly sitting in the waiting room at the local hospital, still waiting to see a doctor.

(Call #12) - As we are getting back into town, we received yet another call. This time there was a twenty-six-year-old male who had forgotten to take his seizure medicine. His fiancée said that he wasn't particularly reliable about taking his prescription medicines as prescribed. We found him lying on his belly in bed. It wasn't hard to arouse our patient from his sleep. In fact he sprang awake and was totally confused. He quickly got to his feet, and appeared he was getting ready to fight. Confusion is always expected after someone experiences a seizure.

He couldn't understand who we were and why we were in his house. Our reluctant patient started storming around in his house, going from room to room cussing and swearing and wanting us to get out and leave him alone. All the while his girlfriend was nearly in a foot race with him, following him into and out of each of the rooms. She was trying, mostly in vain, to make him understand that he just had a grand mal seizure and he was still in a state of confusion. She didn't have any better luck than my partner and I had in trying to reason with him.

Finally he started to come around but now he was getting really belligerent and a little more threatening. Rather than calling the police, I called our medical control (which is the doctor on-duty at the local hospital) and talked to the doctor. I gave him the same information that was given to me by the young man's girlfriend and that I thought that our patient didn't need to be seen. I believed that his fiancée and two other friends who were now at the house would watch over him.

Since our patient was busy stomping around and being really pissed off, I thought better of trying to take a set of vital signs for nothing else other than filling out paperwork. I was relatively certain that he was going to be just fine, providing he takes his medicines more than just once every now and again. The doctor agreed and at 10:52 p.m., we had finished up the call.

11:23 p.m. (Call #13)- I'm not superstitious at all. However, call #13 was certainly unlucky for our next patient. A call came in for a possible gunshot victim. We received this call to back up our other central unit for someone lying in an alley with a gunshot wound to the head. For whatever reason, we arrived at the scene about two minutes before our other unit.

Two city police cars were on scene and when we jumped out of our ambulance, the police officers were already yelling for us to hurry. "He's in bad shape Jim! He's got a head wound!" one of the city cops yelled out.

When we got to the side of unlucky Number 13, he was lying prone (face down) in some icy, snowy slush. I immediately saw a raised area to the middle of the back of his head. After years of experience and dozens and dozens of gunshot wounds to the head, I knew this was an exit wound. We quickly slipped a stiff neck cervical collar around our patient and rolled him over. By this time, the other unit had now arrived on the scene.

As they exited their ambulance, I yelled out to one of the paramedic's, "Bring a backboard and your cot and make it quick! We have a through and through head shot!"

As they got to the side of the patient with their backboard, we slid the patient onto the board and we were able to see that this man in his mid to late twenties had a gunshot entrance wound just above his right eyebrow. His pupils were not dilated but they didn't react to light either. His jaw was clenched so it was impossible to put in endotracheal tube into his airway. Since his breathing was adequate and we were only five to six minutes from the closest emergency room, we elected to put him on a high flow oxygen mask and immediately transported.

While we sped our way to the hospital, I started an IV, reassessed his vital signs and made doubly sure that his breathing was adequate. During our time with him in the ambulance, he was in a decorticate posture. That type of posturing is indicative of a deep and traumatic brain injury. We arrived at the hospital at 11:43 p.m.

From the moment we arrived on scene at the site of the shooting, did our thing, and came through the emergency room doors, it had only been sixteen minutes. Our patient remained a John Doe and laid in bed for more than eight hours, nameless. Just think of it, you're shot in the head and not a single person misses you for more than eight hours.

The on-call neurosurgeon performed surgery later that early morning. A few days later he was still in a vegetative level of consciousness with no real expectation of improvement.

As of this writing, he had been transferred to a long-term care facility.

(Call #14) - While still at the hospital, we were yet dispatched at 12:10 a.m. to another call. There was reportedly a man lying in the street. Since we had one shooting in an alley, it would not have surprised me in the least to see another gun shot victim. We went roaring over to the scene to find a male in his early twenties lying supine in the middle of a side street. He was found by a couple of unrelated people who happened to be walking by. We found him to be conscious, mostly alert and reeking of cheap booze. After checking him over, he had no pain or discernible injuries.

He told us in a very slurred and barely comprehensible speech that he only had six to seven drinks.

After a double take I said to him, "Six or seven! How tall were they?"

Other than making my partner laugh, there was no answer to my inquiring question. All in all, he was just highly intoxicated and a little hypothermic. He wasn't in any danger of dying but had the good citizens not happened by when they did, he most certainly could have. We had him to the hospital at 12:40 a.m., and knocked out the paperwork on our shivering drunkard in only six minutes.

2:57 a.m. (Call #15) - It was one of those kinds of calls that you wish could just wait until 8 a.m. when the oncoming crews would be coming on-duty. It was just a simple return to a nursing home after the patient had made an emergency room visit. The trouble was that the nursing home was halfway across the county.

An 80-year-old man with a history of Alzheimer's disease had just been diagnosed with pneumonia. All of his vital signs were great. The only thing he needed was a little oxygen while we drove him back to the nursing home. By the time we had made it to our destination and had given our report, complete with the all important and pertinent paperwork to the staff at that particular nursing home, it was 3:51 a.m. I had only slept about ninety minutes since beginning my shift at 6:30 a.m. the previous morning.

(Call #16) - We put the cot back into the ambulance and climbed into the front seats, we put ourselves in service. Much to my distress, our dispatcher said, "6511 (our ambulance number), I have another one for you."

You've got to be kidding!

I grabbed our radio microphone and said, "Go ahead with it."
The dispatcher said that we had to see a man with abdominal and left flank pain. To make matters worse it was back across the other side of the county from where we just were. We arrived at the man's house at 4:16 a.m. The local nosy city cops were there and told us that our patient had a history of kidney stones.

This 47-year-old gentleman was in a great deal of pain. He said that he had awakened with excruciating back pain about thirty minutes before he called 911. Furthermore, his pain was now (in addition to his back), in his left flank, abdomen, and the testicular region.

I know from first hand experience how painful kidney stones can be. Pain control is absolutely necessary. Even with that being said, since we were only two miles from the hospital, we elected just to run him over to the emergency room. Had we been twenty minutes or longer away from the hospital, we most likely would have given him enough pain control medicine to buckle his knees.

We finished that call and left the emergency room for the last time, it was at 0445 hours. Fortunately, that was the last ambulance call in our 24-hour shift. Sixteen calls for one ambulance crew is a busy day for us at Medic 1. My personal record is twenty-eight calls.

So let's take a look at this particular day and analyze what had happened and further more, let's see how often an ambulance was actually needed.

We started out the day with a guy who jumped out of his car before it hit a tree. I'll grant you he needs a brain, but right now, that's not the issue. Did he need an ambulance? Answer: Yes.

Call number 2: The lady who had the sharp shooting chest pain while working at the hamburger joint. Did she need an ambulance? Answer: No. What she or anybody else needs to do is to take a couple of breaths before flying off the handle. What would happen if each of us called for an ambulance for some sort of pain before waiting to see whether it would subside by itself?

Call number 3: The lady with spontaneous neck pain who had a bad neck injury months earlier. Did she need an ambulance? Answer: Yes. This reoccurrence of a problem with your neck be it by pain, motor or sensory perception is nothing to fool with.

Call number 4: Take the elderly woman from the emergency room back to her home to be treated by Hospice. Answer: Technically yes. However better coordination and understanding between the family, Hospice and the oncologist would have negated the need for an ambulance in the first place. So the real answer should have been, no.

Call number 5: The lady at the nursing home convalescing from hip surgery with some transient chest pain. Did she need an ambulance? Answer: No. Again, this patient should have been given the opportunity to just relax and see if this pain persisted for even a short period of time. Even though the woman didn't want to go to the hospital, the nurse put undue stress and the ever present "what ifs" in the patient's (and her husband's) mind. The fact of the matter is that first and foremost because of legal issues and liabilities, when an elderly patient complains of chest pain, the nurse will call the doctor and the doctor will almost invariably have her call an ambulance and have them sent to the emergency room.

Call number 6: A woman with cramps to her arms and legs. Did she need an ambulance? Answer: No. The only thing this woman needed was transportation to her local doctor's office, not a hospital. It was a total misuse of EMS that is all too common.

Call number 7: The crack addict who was thrity-one weeks pregnant and complaining of lower abdominal pain. Did she need an ambulance? Answer: Yes. Although this particular patient in my opinion is a piece of human debris, nonetheless, because of her obstetrical history, this call had all of the potential of being an extremely serious medical emergency.

Call number 8: The deputy who rescued the elderly couple from their burning home. Did he need an ambulance? Answer: Yes. Due to his continued respiratory distress, he needed oxygen and follow up at the emergency room.

Call number 9: The woman with stomach pain following a bowel movement. Did she need an ambulance? Answer: No. Of course she didn't. Like so many others, the only thing she needed was a cab ride. As far as I know, most taxicabs don't take Medicaid.

Call number 10: The stupidest call of the day. This was for the old woman at the nursing home that picked at her scab that was over her right eye and caused it to bleed. Did she need an ambulance? Answer: If you don't know, then you too might need to be in a nursing home.

Call number 11: A woman that didn't know who else she should call for her unusual menstruation. Did she need an ambulance? Answer: No. But what can I tell you. She didn't know who to call, so when all else fails (or at least doesn't come to mind), call 911.

Call number 12: A call for the guy in his 20's who had a seizure because he doesn't take his Rx medicines as prescribed. Did he need an ambulance? No. What he needed was a swift kick in the ass for putting himself and everybody else around him at risk. That's not to mention the cost for unnecessary health care because you're too stupid or recalcitrant to take a couple of pills as prescribed.

Call number 13: The gunshot wound to the head of our John Doe. Does he need an ambulance? Answer: Yes. Another true blue, red light emergency!

Call number 14: The drunken putz found lying in the middle of the road. Did he need an ambulance? Answer: Yes. Although he could have just as easily gone home and got into a warm bed and slept it off, he ended up face down on an ice and snow-covered street. Taking him to the hospital to be examined for hypothermic-related injuries was necessary and the prudent thing to do.

Call number 15: Return the old lady to her nursing home at 0351 in the morning. Did she need an ambulance? Answer: Yes. As aggravating as it is at that hour in the morning after running calls for twenty hours, she obviously needed that type of transportation to get her back to her place of residence.

Call number 16: The guy with the kidney stone pain. Did he need an ambulance? Answer: Well, maybe. While it is true that he needed help in the form of pain relief, due to his close proximity to the local hospital (less than two miles), he could have found other transportation.

So let's count them up. As I have it, out of the sixteen times our particular ambulance was summoned for people supposedly in need, in reality our services were only required seven times. Of the other nine times (one being a definite "maybe"), there were a wide variety of reasons why, but in the final analysis, we weren't really needed. What this amounts to is that nine out of sixteen ambulance calls were a general waste of services, time and usually taxpayer-sponsored money.

This twenty-four hour stretch we were needed as EMS providers more than most days. It was a long, grueling shift filled with a variety of problems and some adventure. For a few of the patients we did some good and eased a little pain and anxiety. For two elderly patients, we provided medically required transportation. The majority of our calls were as a "taxi service" to provide simple transportation to the hospital. The plain truth of the matter, this was just another day.

Chapter 15
NUTS AND JOLTS

The following are several short stories that are remarkable for the humor it elicited by the ambulance crews that were on the scene at the time. They are but a small fraction of the crazy and zany things that have happened when paramedics and EMT's cross paths with the local, over-stressed ding-a-lings and dimwits. Admittedly, not all of the following will be seen as being particular funny or humorous by everyone.

There is a certain "coffin humor" when it comes to this type of profession. It's just that sometime you may not know whether you should laugh or cry, sympathize or scold, intervene or let the nature of people play itself out. The people who work as professionals in this business or those who volunteer their time and talents see so much pain and suffering. We see everything from natural causes as well as causes born of either violence or stupidity that you really have to find humor whenever and however you can.

I will admit that I show a certain lack of respect to some people. Those types of people I show disdain toward are for those who use the emergency services for—as they see it—their "free" taxi ride to the hospital for non-existent or near non-existent medical problems. Those that misuse, willfully abuse, and think that I owe them a living, are fair game for ridicule, mockery, scorn and above all.........laughter. Right or wrong, it's how I keep my sanity in an all too often, insane world.

***

A call came in for me on a spring evening at about 9 p.m., to see a man who thought that he might "have to die." I quickly recognized the address of this particular call as being at the apartment building of a man who occasionally called for EMS help. But knowing this particular man as I do, I know that he's harmless enough and he just usually needs a little bit of reassurance that there isn't anyone in his closet or under his bed. Or, that he isn't sick and above all, doesn't need to go to the local hospital.

This guy is really a nice man in his mid to late 40s, who doesn't have a malicious bone in his body. The fact of the matter is that Ned lived by himself and was mentally a little slow. At the same time we were dispatched and took our subsequent leisurely drive to take care of Ned, my current partner, Jed Tiller and I had a third, ride along. Cody Phillips was currently working in our wheel-chair division and was looking to advance into the ambulance side of our ambulance company.

Medic 1 allows prospective employees who eventually want to work for the ambulance side of the company to ride "third" so the duty crew members can assess their capabilities, work ethic, as well as their strengths and weaknesses. This also allows the third rider to see and get a "good feel" about the ambulance business and the advanced life support side of EMS. Sometimes it turns out to be a match made in heaven and sometimes...not.

We got to Ned's apartment building and knocked on the door. In a somewhat soft voice, he said, "Come on in." We enter to find him sitting on a chair at his small kitchen table looking somewhat socially withdrawn and pensive.

He didn't appear to be in any kind of physical pain or acute distress, so I said to him, "What's up Ned? Why did you call us today?"

With a certain resignation in his voice he says to me, "I think I might have to die."

Knowing that our dispatcher had given only that small bit of information to us I wasn't surprised with his answer but I could hardly wait for his reason as to why he thought his demise was imminent.

"What do you mean, 'you might have to die.'"

"I just got out of church and they said I couldn't eat or drink for forty days."

As I looked at him I could see he had a very small "+" sign in the middle of his forehead. It was then that I remembered that today was Ash Wednesday.

As I continued my questioning I said, "Who said you couldn't eat or drink anything for forty days?"

"The priest said that."

"No Ned, the priest didn't say that. You must have misunderstood what he was saying or trying to say."

Ned suddenly continued in a near frantic tone and said, "No! He said we couldn't eat or drink for forty days!"

Trying to calm Ned down I said back to him, "Listen to me Ned. What the priest meant was that you couldn't drink alcohol, you know beer and booze and that kind of thing. That's what he was trying to tell you. And as far as not eating, let me assure you that nobody and especially Jesus doesn't expect you not to eat for forty days either."

With a huge sigh of relief, Ned says back to me, "Do you really think so?"

"Certainly Ned, I know so. You see that stack of empty pizza boxes sitting on the floor next to your refrigerator? (There were about a dozen of them) You should give up pizza for forty days. Jesus just might like that. Besides, it'll be good for you as well."

Ned ponders for a moment what I was trying to get across to him and I could tell his "gears were turning" in respect to what I had just said.

He then looked at me earnestly straight in the eye and replied, "Are you giving up anything?"

Without missing a beat I said, "Well Ned, I'm not Catholic but my wife informs me that I'll be giving up sex for the next forty days and so is Cody here. Jed's case is a little bit different. Jed, here, is giving up masturbation for 40 days. Isn't that right Jed?"

Without hesitation Jed blurts out, "Hell yes!"

Jed and especially Cody who are both in their early 20's couldn't believe I just said that and as a result, tried really hard not to laugh and each of them turned about six shades of red. Cody was trying not to laugh so hard that I thought he just might wet himself. Seeing their reaction to what I just said made me laugh right out loud. (I know better than to try to keep that bottled up inside).

Anyway before you knew it, the three of us were falling all over ourselves with laughter. "Ned" didn't quite grasp what was said and didn't quite know why we were laughing so hard. Suffice to say, he was just immensely relieved that he didn't have to die after all.

Over the years and perhaps a dozen or more times of Ned calling EMS for help, he has never incurred my wrath at all. The difference is that although Ned is somewhat mentally handicapped, he is gainfully employed (which means he tries hard). Equally important, he doesn't "use" EMS as a means of simple transportation, but calls for help for what he sees as real health related problems. The compassion I feel for someone like Ned is real and heartfelt.

Is he a royal pain sometimes? Yes. Has that ever caused me to disrespect him or others like him that may fall short of societal expectations? Not a chance.

***

Not too often will you find that a car wreck where people were hurt, and property was damaged that turns out to be funny. But sometimes things happen with bystanders that are just hilarious. Such was the case where at the time my good friend and partner Ed Witucki and I were dispatched for a car accident in an inner-city neighborhood. Since it wasn't too far from our central station, Ed and I arrived at the accident scene three to four minutes before the police.

The trouble was that about sixty people arrived before we did. When Ed and I climbed out of our ambulance, we climbed into a highly chaotic scene that bordered on being violent. We found that there were several groups of people who were in extremely heated arguments.

What had happened was that a scoundrel, who was driving a car, had an under aged, mentally-challenged person performing a sex act on him while he was driving. He lost control of his car and drove through a couple of residential yards. During his brief off-road foray, he sideswiped two cars before slamming into a third.

As Ed and I waded through the crowd of people on our way to where the supposed injured man was located, we could easily hear the verbal threats being aimed at the man who had been driving his car. As it turned out, a few of the people whose property had been damaged by this rogue had not so gently removed him from his car and were just on the verge of kicking the hell out of this guy when Ed and I arrived at his side.

When Ed and I got to where the man had been pulled from his car, we found him sitting on the ground, leaning against his wrecked car, with his pants pulled down. With what we were hearing from the crowd, on our way to this man's side, it didn't surprise me to find him partially nude.

About the only thing I could think to say in disgust to Ed was, "Oh for Christ's sake Ed, look at this idiot! And he even has his lizard hanging out."

That must have struck Ed as being really funny because he started to laugh really hard.

By this time, the local city police department was on site with several officers and they had just started to get the accident scene under control by moving the people back and out of the way. As I further evaluated our patient's injuries, Ed had gone back to our ambulance to retrieve our cot, along with a backboard and cervical collar.

By the time my partner was back with the needed equipment, I had finished assessing our patient's condition and found him appearing heavily intoxicated. Other than being slightly bruised along with a few scrapes, he appeared that he was essentially unhurt, which would not have been the case had Ed and I arrived two minutes later than we did.

In just a few short minutes we had fitted our patient with a cervical collar, placed him on our backboard and lifted him onto our ambulance cot. At this time it became apparent that the mother of the child that this man had in his car was now at the accident scene and found out what had happened. To say the least, she understandably was just a little more than upset. The fact was that she was furious and was just raising all kinds of hell.

She was a large woman. She was maybe, at the most five-feet-four inches tall and weighing in excess of 350 pounds. She was cussing and swearing at this guy at the top of her lungs and made several attempts to get a piece of him by attempting to go through the police lines. Finally, one of the officers told her that she would find herself under arrest if she interfered further.

That must have struck a chord with her because although she could have shot daggers through this rogue with her eyes, she said nothing more and remained behind the police tape. She just stood on her feet, rocking back and forth at the police line with her pursed lips and searing eyes. It was obvious to me that she was just barely able to emotionally and physically keep herself under control.

As Ed and I lifted the backboard with our patient onto our cot, we secured the patient with the restraining straps and started to wheel the cot toward our ambulance. As luck would have it, we had to go right next to where this woman was anxiously standing. Ed had the foot end of the cot and was pulling, and I had the head end and was pushing. As we neared the area to where the mad mama bear was standing, I had an instant idea.

(As a note, I have almost always been in favor of instant justice.) With that in mind, I pulled back on our cot as to bring it almost to a complete stop. Just as I thought, this woman reached out and slapped this guy in the face as hard as she could—not once, not twice, but eight times.

Of course I then stepped up acting all indignant and said, "Okay lady, okay, that's enough! That's enough!"

As I pushed the cot past to where this woman had just gotten her own kind of justice, Ed looked at me like I had just lost my mind. Without Ed saying a word to me and as I looked back at him, I said, "What? She needed that and he richly deserved it. I don't have a problem with it at all."

Ed quickly turns around from me, so the only thing I can see is his back. After knowing Ed for more than twenty-five years, I can tell by his body language that he's just laughing his ass off.

As we approached the ambulance, Ed had to look at me again. His face was red with tears of laughter.

I then looked down at this guy as we are just getting ready to load him into our ambulance and sternly said to him, "And if you hit me, I'm going to call that woman whose kid you had in your car and I'll have her kill you right here and right now! You got that?"

Without a second to think about it, the mook on our cot says to Ed and me, "Oh hell no! Take me to jail! Just take me to jail right now!"

As Ed and I are just starting to bust a gut over his pitiful pleading as to not let this woman get at him again, I said to him, "Don't worry buddy. You're heading there sooner than you think."

***

A few minutes later, we left the scene as we had just remanded our would-be patient back over to the police department. As we are leisurely driving back to our central station, Mike is still doubled-over with laughter over the whole incident.

He said to me, "Stine, if you could have seen your own face when you realized it wasn't a gunshot wound, you'd be laughing too. Goddamn, it was precious! And then when you told him to pull his punk-ass pants up and get the hell out of the ambulance (now Mike is laughing so hard I can't hardly understand him), I thought I might just piss myself!"

A couple of years later Mike and I were discussing that call again. As usual Mike started laughing about it again.

He turned to me and said, "I'm telling you what Stine. As I someday draw my last breath that will be one of the last things I'll be remembering."

***

One of the more irritating things to have to put with is people who use us for nothing more than a mode for convenient (and free to them) transportation. What's worse is this abuse is perpetrated by many people. But the thing that makes it worse yet, is the fact that about a dozen or so of those people call us all of the time! And let's be clear, it's never for anything of any substance, let alone a bona fide emergency.

A few years ago we had one of those days where in the course of our usual twenty-four hour shift, we were getting hammered. I mean it was one call after another, after another, after another. It was one of those days where the vast majority of the calls were true emergencies. I remember nobody had a chance to eat any meals at all, at least not until close to midnight.

Usually by that time, I am just too tired to eat anything more than a snack or some such thing. I have to also admit that when I'm that tired, I don't play so well with others. Consequently, I'm not adequately able to tolerate our "frequent flyer club" members when they call us to "come and check me out" or "it's three o'clock in the morning and I need to go to the hospital because I've had a cough and running nose for the last ten days and right now, it's an emergency.

One of our frequent flyers Denny, starts calling. The first call was just prior to midnight. As my partner, Dave Hawkins and I arrived, we found him lying in the middle of his small front yard acting like he had been shot. As it turned out, he was out drinking himself into oblivion and his liver or something was letting him know about it.

The first thing he said to us was, "Hey man, you gotta help me. I need to go to the hospital. I'm sick and I gotta go."

"Of course you're sick, you moron. As often as you swim in that cheap rotgut slop you drink, I'm surprised you don't have gills and fins by now! Denny, just what in the hell do you expect us or the hospital staff to do for you. It's obvious you don't give a damn about yourself and you don't want to help yourself at all either, unless it is of course to get shit-faced each and every day!"

As expected, Denny is about as mad as he can be. The last thing he wants of course is to be lectured about his lifestyle and to be told to get his act together. He doesn't want us to insist that he act like a man and quit bothering us for nothing more than an ordinary cab ride to the local hospital. But of course the little show continues.

"Fine, just leave me alone then. Just let me die right here!"

"Oh c'mon, Denny. What do you mean die? Saying that just means your trying to tease us. Please Denny, I'm too tired for teasing, so if you're going to die, please, you just go right ahead. Believe me, I won't mind a bit."

He screamed back at me, "I know you don't care if I die, you bastard!"

"Now, now Denny, let's not call each other names. You just be a good boy and lay there and die if you want to."

He looks up from the dirt, weeds and bugs and said, "Just get the hell out of here."

"Denny, no sooner said than done. See 'ya."

Dave and I quickly spun around and briskly walked back to our ambulance and drove back to our station. The whole episode took us about fifteen minutes. As we got back to the station, parked the ambulance and got back into the crew quarters, it was about 12:30 a.m. After running nearly solid from 8 a.m. the previous morning until now, I was more than ready to have some down time. Well, that lasted less than an hour.

The other crew at the stationed had just been sent to another call when our dispatch center received a call from Denny, telling us that he was complaining about vomiting up blood. Honestly speaking, some long-time alcoholics do develop a condition that renders the blood vessels in their esophagus very fragile, becoming like varicose veins.

When one of those breaks or ruptures, it can be a life threatening event. In this particular case I've known Denny for years and I know he's never had that condition. Tonight, it's just his latest rendition of whining, crying and feeling sorry for himself. But nonetheless, we drive over to Denny's house (again) and I remember muttering to Dave something about, if he wasn't bleeding out of his mouth when we arrived, that he's going to be bleeding out of his nose when we left!

As we arrived at his house again after only being away less than an hour, from the ambulance I could see Denny lying face down on his front porch. I turned to Dave and said in disgust, "Oh look at Denny. He's made it another twenty-five feet from his yard to his porch. Now he's face down again. Ain't this a bitch?"

As Dave and I rolled to a stop, I grabbed my flashlight and walked across the small yard. I walked up the three or four porch steps to where he was pretending to need our services, again.

"Denny, what's the trouble now? Why are you bothering my partner and me again? Other than having an acute allergy to gainful employment and being a major league pain in the ass to society at large, just what in the hell is your major malfunction today?"

"Like I said, I'm vomiting blood!" he screamed.

"Listen Denny, don't you start yelling at us!" As I shined the light on the pool of stomach contents that he is now laying his face in, I said to him, "Denny, there's not a single drop of your blood in that mess your lying in. It's just a wild mixture of the cheapest, nastiest bunch of rotgut swill you could pour into yourself.

"But the last thing you want for us to do is see you again tonight. So get your sorry ass off the porch and get in the ambulance. Dave and I along with all of the other fine taxpaying people who work for a living are going to give your sorry ass a ride to the hospital. I know the staff there can't wait to see you.......again."

Without looking up at either of us he mumbles and says, "I can't walk and I pay taxes too."

Dave then said to him, "If you can't walk, you can't ride. Denny, there is a zero chance that Jim and I are going to carry your ass anywhere! Besides taxes on beer and cheap wine doesn't count as paying taxes, you asshole!"

For some reason, I don't know why, but that last remark by Dave just got me laughing my ass off. Maybe I was by this time a little too over stressed or too fatigued, because if I didn't start to laugh, I might just give Denny that bloody nose I was talking about earlier.

As I was busy falling all over myself, Denny looked up at the two of us with the emesis dripping off of his face and says, "Fuck you guys. I'll just lay here all night."

"Go ahead and lay there. But I'm telling you, Denny, I'm at my limit with you. I don't want to see you again. I don't want you to call us again. You've plainly worn everybody out with your stupidity and we are all sick and tired of it. So do yourself a favor and don't call us again."

I honestly, foolishly, thought, that would be the last we would be hearing from him—or at the least, that night. How dumb was that thinking? When we arrived back at our station, we told the other duty crew that we just got back from Denny's house for the second time in as many hours. We told them how we had found him the first time and how he had made it to his porch before calling us a second time. After describing his condition in which we found him the second time, our two colleagues who also knew Denny as well as anybody, started laughing.

Then I said, "Yeah, Denny informed us that he paid taxes just like everybody else did. But then Dave went ahead and busted his bubble by telling him that taxes on his rot gut liquor didn't count."

Then our two buddies really started laughing. We all went back to bed and within a few minutes the other crew received a call for a shooting. They scrambled out of the station and were gone in no time at all.

I called out to my partner, "Ya' know, that's just great isn't it? They get a call for a shooting and we get Denny not once but twice!"

We made small talk and then quickly drifted off to a well-earned sleep.

About thirty minutes later I picked up the ringing phone, "Yes?"

With a heavy sigh the dispatcher said to me, "Jim, I hate to have to tell you this but…" I cut him off in mid sentence and said, "Don't tell me that Denny wants to see us again?"

"Yes he does," our dispatcher quietly responded.

"Well that's just it! I'm going to go over there and jerk a knot in his tail!"

I hung up the phone and my partner Dave was already getting dressed and was grumbling about being used as a convenient taxicab for nothing but lizards and scumbags. So once again we drove the three or four minutes to Denny's house. Seeing that he no longer was taking up space in the yard or on his front porch we entered his house through the front door and found Denny casually sitting on a kitchen chair with his legs crossed just smoking a cigarette. Not surprisingly, he didn't look like he was in any distress at all.

Without asking him anything, I just started yelling at him, "What in the hell is your problem now? Why are we here for the third time in less than three hours? Do you think we are here for your every wish and whim? What is wrong with your wine-soaked brain anyway?!"

He answers me in almost in a matter-of-fact tone and said, "Man, my stomach is really bothering me. I think I'll be alright, if I can get something to eat."

For a moment the three of us just stared at each other. I guess Dave and I were really trying to process what he wanted from us this time around.

I immediately put my hand to my chest in a gesture of disbelief and exclaimed, "Do you expect us to fix you something to eat at three o'clock in the morning?! Have you completely lost your mind!? Where is it written, spoken or even thought that you should call EMS to cook your breakfast?!" I'm literally screaming at him "What in the hell is wrong with you?!"

He yells right back at me and unbelievably said, "It's your job to help me and I need help getting something to eat!" "You're supposed to do your job, that's what you're supposed to do!"

I know he's serious and as a result I'm simply just speechless. I know that I'm dead-dog tired, but how does one argue with that kind of logic?

"Denny, we are under no circumstances cooking you breakfast and furthermore you're not calling us again!"

With that I saw where his wall-mounted phone was located. As I walked over to it, I drew my fist back and swung at it as hard as I could and punched it clean off of the wall. It was one of those old-fashioned big wall-mounted phones with a huge plastic base. After my fist struck the phone, there were phone parts lying all over the place. The only thing left on the wall was the metal mounting bracket and the phone wire.

"Denny" gets up off of the kitchen chair in a huff and walks sternly toward me clearly angry and said, "Man, you just wrecked my phone!"

In complete agreement, I said back to him in a very calm voice and said, "Yes I did. But think of it this way Denny that was going to be either your phone or your nose. If I were you, I'd count my blessings and I'd also take a few steps back."

With that, Dave and I walked past Denny and left his house. We returned back to our station chuckling over the whole "Denny" episode. It was great to be able to laugh, because while we were at his house, we were clearly fresh out of humor.

***

Another one of my more entertaining frequent flyers, was for a woman who was clearly a hypochondriac. She was a 40-plus-year-old, and was probably at least 200 pounds over weight. She was always complaining about a cough and cold, some obscure pain in one of her arms or legs, or some other dire emergency. She would call us for the most vague, indistinct, and self-contrived complaints that you could imagine.

I remember several of her "imagined emergencies." Complaints such as "my elbow hurts when I bend it." "My eyes are twitching." "I think my ankle is swollen." "I keep having gas." Well, after weeks of this kind of requests for an ambulance turn to months, I generally have the propensity to become a little testy over this kind of complaint.

One day, we were called to respond for the umpteenth time to Lena's house. It was for her usual, ridiculous, and absurd complaint about her elbow hurting whenever she bends it. I had had enough.

"Lena, don't you realize just how trivial 'arm pain' is? Do you honestly think that you should call paramedics for simple, non-traumatic arm pain? Do you honestly think that you should go to a hospital for this kind of pain? Why would you think that you couldn't or shouldn't take a couple of aspirin to get rid of your arm pain? What would make you think that you need the emergency services of para-medics?"

She responded, "Well go on! If you don't want to help me, just get out of my house!" She started to literally cry. "You just don't care about me! Just get out! Get out!"

"Now Lena, nobody is saying that they don't care about you. But the fact of the matter is that whenever you call us, we all know it's for a bunch of crap. Whenever I get sent over here, I know it's going to be because your feet are sore or you have a headache or some other idiotic complaint and quite frankly, I'm sick of it. You can cry and scream and yell all you want. We are here to help those that NEEEEED our help, not for elbow pain, sore feet or whatever else you dream up."

"Lena" screams back at me, "Don't you talk to me that way! You can't say that to me!"

"Oh yes I can!" I said and now I'm raising my voice, "Quit your damn crying because I'm not buying that either. Just get up and get into the ambulance. I don't want to hear anything else you have to say because I know it's just a load of crap!"

Suddenly she quit crying and just as fast, started moving her elbow back and forth like she trying to fan herself. "My elbow really does hurt, damn it!"

Now I'm yelling back to her, "Well the way you're moving it, it can't hurt that bad. Besides, I don't care that your elbow hurts Lena. That's not the point. The point is that you shouldn't be calling us for this bullshit in the first place!"

Lena started tearing up again. I told her, "Why is that so hard for you to understand? Nobody cares that you have a headache that you won't even take an aspirin for. Nobody cares that your feet are sore because you're carrying around a half ton of weight; all the while you are stuffing your face full of donuts!

"Nobody cares about that kind of complaint because nobody can help that except for you! Instead, you want us to take you to the hospital so the nurses can hold your hand and tell you that you'll be all right and the doctor can tell you that all is well. Well let me tell you, nobody has time for that anymore. The fact of the matter is that you are just wearing everybody out!"

Now she was really blubbering, "Just get out of my house you bastards! Get out! Get out!" she screamed.

"Hey Lena, no sooner said than done. See ya'!" I yelled back at her.

The very next day that I'm working, Lena calls again. This time I happened to be sitting in the dispatch office.

The dispatcher turns to me and asks, "Are you ready for this? There is a female complaining of just wanting an ambulance. She couldn't or wouldn't tell me any more than that."

I said to her, "That's Lena's house. For God's sake, what does she want with us now?" Our dispatcher said back to me, "Apparently, she wants you to take her to the hospital."

By this time, this whole daily routine is getting both bothersome and humorous. So, without further ado, my partner, Ryan Cronk and I hop into our ambulance and take a leisurely drive over to her house. Once we are there, we knock on her door and walk into her living room.

Building on our last encounter I said to her, "What's it this time Lena? Why do you think you need an ambulance today?

She depicts some sort of vague, idiotic pain that she really can't describe. She said something about being tired and doesn't have any energy or some such song and dance.

As Lena is rambling on, I interrupted her and asked, "Lena", pardon me for asking the obvious, but did you buy any chance at all just happen to call your doctor and ask him about your lack of energy? Did you ever consider doing at least, that?"

Immediately Lena starts blubbering and wailing away.

I turned to my partner and said, "Ryan, I can't believe this bullshit. This is the same crap she pulled with me just two days ago." As I turned toward Lena I started yelling at her, mostly because she was doing her "crying" so loud, I wasn't sure she would hear me if I didn't yell. "Stop this crying! Do you hear me Lena? I said stop this crying act! We're not buying this idiotic crying routine of yours!"

While still blubbering at the top of her lungs, she yells to Ryan and me, "Get out! I don't want you here!"

She then gets up from her chair. While she is screaming and crying, she walks out of her house and goes across the street and cries to her neighbors. I couldn't believe it. I turned to Ryan half pissed off, half bewildered and totally amused and just shrugged my shoulders.

Ryan said to me, "Well since she left the scene, I guess we no longer have a patient."

I have to admit, it did sound funny to me. "That sounds great to me Cronk buddy. Let's go before she changes her mind." We left her house and didn't hear back from her again for the rest of the day.

The very next time I am working, "Lena" calls yet again. Although I wasn't "up" for the next call, I told the dispatcher that Ryan and I would take the call. I figured that this was going to be a hoot. As we rolled up to the shoulder of the road in front of her house, she was sitting on a chair on her front porch. As we came to a stop, she stood up and when she saw me get out of the front seat of the ambulance and although I was probably forty feet from her and hadn't uttered a word her way, she started her screaming and crying routine again.

From more than thirty feet from me she yells out, "I don't want you! You're a bad man! I want somebody else!"

I yelled back to her, "Well you're not getting anybody else! You don't get to decide who comes here to give you your free ride!"

She refused to go with us and was already on the phone asking for another ambulance crew to come and take her to the hospital. Our dispatcher, Karen was excellent at her duties. As I got on the radio to talk to her, she put Lena on hold. I told Karen, that if Lena called again, to tell her that Ryan and I would be the crew to take her to the hospital.

Karen knew all too well about Lena's history. To that end she quickly took her off of hold and then proceeded to tell her that, "If you need an ambulance again, Mr. Stine will be the paramedic to come and get you and he wanted me tell you that he will be more than glad to see you again."

Once Ryan and I got back to our central station we went to our dispatch center to see Karen. She was already laughing.

"So what did Lena have to say after hearing that you were going to send Ryan and me back over to her?"

Karen said, "The only thing she said before hanging up the phone on me was…BLAHHHH!"

***

So tell me, what do you do if you have an unwanted person in your house who refuses to leave? Call the local police department, right? Well, maybe. What do you do if you have an unwanted person who has knee pain and refuses to leave your home? Call the local police department, right? Wrong! Call EMS.

Now, take into consideration that we have absolutely no law enforcement powers whatsoever. Yet my partner, Bill Boyd and I were called to a house at about four o'clock in the morning for someone with "knee pain." As usual I'm slightly annoyed at the trivial nature of the call that could and in all likelihood, should wait until normal day light hours of business.

Nonetheless, we get out of bed, get in the ambulance and drive over to where we were dispatched. We knocked on the door and an elderly woman answered. She said that she, along with her very elderly and infirm husband wanted this other woman out of their house.

To say the least, we were a little mystified as to why we were called as opposed to the local police. The elderly woman said that they had let her into their home earlier in the evening for a hot meal because they felt sorry for her. Apparently things for whatever reason went south relatively fast and they asked her to leave their home. Now for the last several hours, they were having no success in getting her to leave. She and her husband had stayed up all night because they thought, if they retired for the evening, and left her alone in the house, that the unwanted woman would "rob them blind."

I asked the woman why she didn't call the police? She said that she did call the police, but somehow during the call and the ensuing back-and-forth conversation with the police, it was discovered that the unwanted guest had some sort of (contrived) knee pain. So instead of the police department sending a squad car over to get things sorted out, they said she needed EMS.

At any rate, the local police who should have handled this complaint contacted our dispatch center and before you know it, we were on our way over to take care of the problem. This brief and somewhat bewildering conversation between Bill, me and the elderly woman was held right near the front door of this aged couple's house.

Although we still didn't quite "get it," I told the lady to show us to the patient. She led us into the next room and there reclining in a chair is one of our better known frequent fliers.

"Rita! What are you doing here and bothering these nice people?" I said in a most incredulous tone. "These people want you out of their home. Get up off of the chair and get out!"

She turned to me and said, "I can't walk. My knee hurts."

Bill and I had known Rita for years and years and she was a well-known nasty alcoholic and drug abuser who has been in and out of jail over the span of many years from an array of charges. As far as Bill and I are concerned as well as all of our colleagues at Medic 1 who see her regularly, is that she generally only complains of being "sick." And that was usually from drinking the night before. However, tonight its manufactured knee pain that she hoped would keep her in this very nice and older couple's house…or at the least a warm and clean hospital bed.

Bill asks "Rita", "How did you get here?"

"I walked as far as I could and now I can't walk any further." she says.

Bill says in a matter of fact tone, "Well Rita, if you can't walk, you can't ride. It's just as simple as that."

She then says to the both of us, "I'm telling y'all, I can't walk. I need to ride on the ambulance bed!"

At that moment, I cut her off at the pass. "Rita, we've been down this road many times before and you know you're not going to be getting on our cot. Like Bill just said, if you're not going to walk, you're not going to ride. And when we leave, we'll be calling the police and they will come over and throw you out of this house. So make up your mind, is it us or is it the police?"

With that, Bill turned around and started heading toward the front door. As I turned to follow my partner, I said, "We're leaving Rita. Goodbye Rita."

Almost at once, she started cussing and carrying on about this and that, and all the while complaining and insisting that she couldn't walk at all. Of course by now she is up and out of the chair limping our way. As I walked past the elderly woman, I quickly told her that once we have Rita out of the house that she should shut and lock the door behind us. She nodded in agreement.

As I exited the front door, I saw that Bill was already curb side and in the back of the ambulance with the side doors wide open. Rita was still complaining about her knee pain, even though I could plainly see she was hardly limping at all.

Finally I said to her, "Quit your bitching and just keep moving. We can look at your knee once we get into the back of the ambulance."

Bill then calls out to her, "C'mon Rita, get your ass in here."

With that she stopped just outside the ambulance door and proclaims, "Y'all just want to see my pussy!"

I was aghast! Seeing her perpetually drunk, smelling as though she didn't believe in bathing more than once a season, her foul language and demeanor, apparently wasn't enough.

After hearing her last comment, I just spun around and said, "Rita, you are a disgusting creature and a disgrace to your race!"

She immediately yelled back, "Race? I ain't been in no race. I just gots me out of jail this morning!"

I just shook my head, and headed toward the driver's side of the ambulance. Bill was laughing so hard that he was literally in tears, and could hardly walk. He did all he could just climbing out of the patient compartment through the side doors.

Rita just stood there on the sidewalk watching Bill get into the front passenger seat. As he slammed the passenger door shut, I inched the ambulance slowly from the curb and onto the street. She started walking along side the ambulance still insisting that she couldn't walk; still proclaiming her need to go to the hospital. With all of that, she also started yelling, cussing and hurling all kinds of insults.

Ever so slowly, I increased the speed of the ambulance. "Rita" was now briskly walking...then jogging...then, eventually flat out running. This took no longer than perhaps thirty seconds. All the while through his laughter, Bill was cheering her on, and waving for her to keep up with the ambulance.

As Bill and I were watching her flat out run, and then finally fade into the pre-dawn darkness, we figured we had cured her knee pain. If not, we were sure that we had alleviated the pain a little further up the back of the leg that the elderly couple had been feeling all night long.

Chapter 16
THE ENEMY WITHIN

Most of the preceding events were either funny at the time in which they occurred, or a short time later when the call could be viewed in retrospect. Unfortunately, that is not always the case. Once in a while, there is someone who is legitimately, mentally ill. I'm not talking about those who have a flash crisis that may involve a teenager who broke up with his or her boyfriend or girlfriend. Nor the "I had a big fight with my mother and I hate her guts because she grounded me for a month" routine.

With those types of ambulance calls I usually get involved because on many occasions the aggrieved person (who is now my patient) has locked him or herself into the bathroom threatening to end it all. Invariably, they are screaming through the locked door their intentions to either overdose themselves with prescription medication or cut themselves with a razor blade. Typically, my partner and I will try to talk to them through the door, tell them that they have to come out and be medically evaluated, and most likely will now have to go to the local hospital because they threatened suicide.

Usually the person relinquishes and comes out uninjured, and ready to talk it out. Once in a while, we'll have to threaten to kick the door down and drag them out. Rarely do we (or the attending police department) have to break in a door and get physical with someone, but it has happened. It's been my experience that the vast majority of these patients are in a state of raging anger as evidenced by screaming out a highly colorful array of language about some social injustice "unfairly" perpetrated on them by either a relative, friend, lover or neighbor. This type of call simply does not interest me.

What I speak of are those who have a true psychosis. It's about those few individuals who through no fault of their own are hallucinating, delusional, or might have a true distortion or complete break from reality. As viewed through the prism of a longtime EMS provider most of these patients can be categorized into two groups.

The first group is the ego systonic or smiling set of patients. Though they may be totally clueless of who they are, where they're at or what they are doing, they present themselves as happy or pleasantly content. They are rarely if ever a danger or menace to themselves or anyone else. It may not sound nice, but the possible entertainment value of these types of patients more often than not becomes readily apparent. I, along with many others in EMS, actually look forward to interacting with the happy patients that have escaped reality.

An example of a patient that had an ego systonic psychosis, was when my partner Bob Ristau and I were called to the emergency room of our local hospital. After our arrival and subsequent discussion with the hospital nursing and medical staff, we were introduced to a female in her mid-40s who was resting comfortably. She had a pleasant demeanor and wasn't sure what all the fuss was about and why she was wasting time lying around in the emergency room.

According to the nursing staff, her family became alarmed when she awoke that morning asking who was going to drive her from her home in Chicago, Illinois to her nightclub act in Milwaukee, Wisconsin. One problem was that she had always lived in southwest Michigan and had never resided in Chicago. Another problem was that she didn't then, nor did she ever have an entertainment career of any kind. But according to her, she was a nightclub singer eagerly awaiting a ride to her next performance.

Feeling certain that she wouldn't be too keen on the idea of having us take her to a psychiatric hospital in Kalamazoo, MI and as not to distress her, I told her that Bob and I were called to make sure she got to Milwaukee in short order. When we got her into the ambulance for an approximately one-hour ride to the psychiatric hospital, I had a pleasant and fascinating conversation with her for the first ten minutes of our trip.

I quizzed her on things like: How long have you been a singer? Are you a solo artist or do you have a band? What style of music or genre do you sing? Where and how often do you sing? The questions went on for almost ten minutes and she answered every one of them with an aura of self-confidence and a true belief in her abilities. I was astounded because I knew for certain that all of this was pure fantasy. Yet, I also knew for certain that in her mind it was an absolute matter of fact.

I didn't know it at the time, but my second to the last question to her of what is your favorite song to sing, would trigger a performance.

And what a performance it would be! She told me it was "Strangers in the Night", her signature song. She said she was well known for it in not only Milwaukee, but also in Sheboygan and Green Bay, Wisconsin.

"Do you want to hear it? I did it with Frank Sinatra!" she asked with much excitement.

With a big smile and an answer that I would regret for the next forty minutes and then later laugh about, I said, "Sure. If you did it with ol' blue eyes, I'd love to hear it."

For some reason, I started with fascination to buy in to her delusional notion that she perhaps was a singer. I know it sounds ridiculous, but the way she answered the questions I posed to her with a hint of swagger and boasting of her many fans and how booked-up she was, was incredible. Then she started singing.

*"Strangers in the night exchanging glances…
Wond'ring in the night what were the chances…
We'd be sharing love before the night was through…
Something in your eyes was so inviting…
Something in your smile was so exciting…
Something in my heart told me I must have you…"*

This went on non-stop for about forty minutes and to say it sounded like fingernails on a chalkboard would be kind.

My last question would be repeated several times. "Can you sing something else or perhaps give it a rest?" (It would soon become obvious that "give it a rest" was never going to be a consideration.)

"Yes, I can sing something else."

Each time she would hesitate for three to four seconds as if she was thinking or deciding on her next song selection. After her choice was made she would reposition herself on the ambulance bench seat in which was sitting, clear her throat, methodically wet her lips and finally her eyes would quickly dart from her left to her right as if she was checking her audience.

And then she would start singing, *"Strangers in the night exchanging glances..."* and on it went again and again.

As she started her third rendition, Bob started to sing loudly with her. Then I joined in to make it a trio. Following our patient's lead, Bob and I sang each recital with more gusto than the last. During our time together the lead crooner in our group momentarily lost her focus three different times while singing and would forget the words to our only musical piece. With just a brief hint of hesitation she would fall back on the song's closing refrain and belt out, *"Shoo-be, do-be-do.....la-da-da-da....."*

Each time that happened, Bob and I would quickly follow her lead no matter where it took us. As we arrived and rolled to a stop at the psychiatric hospital, Bob and I thanked her for allowing us to sing with her. We walked her into the facility and turned her over to the specialized staff.

As I turned to her to bid her adieu she asked me, "Will I see you guys at one of my shows?"

"We will definitely catch you on your tour," I said.

"Connie, we wouldn't miss it for the world," Bob added.

With the last word she said, "Okay, I'll see you guys then."

Anyone with a minimal amount of hearing let alone any musical appreciation would never have had to differentiate the three of us from Peter, Paul and Mary, but we had a genuinely great and memorable time.

I don't know how our patient ever turned out. I wish I did. And although she was obviously delusional, she was also one of the most self-assured people I have ever had as a psychiatric patient. I hope she responded positively to the mental healthcare she needed.

***

Unfortunately, the second group is much more prevalent than the ego systonic patients. They are the "ego dystonic" or unpleasant patients. They are the aggressive and unpredictable men and women whose psychosis lends itself to irrational violence and who truly believe that their death is imminent and therefore have a real and palpable fear for their lives.

With the mentally ill patients who fit the category of ego dystonic psychosis comes the sheer pain and agony and sometimes the human tragedy in which such an illness strikes; and often with such devastating consequences.

A couple of years ago I was assigned to be working at an outlying station with my partner, Nate, when we received a call from our EMS dispatcher. We were told that our ambulance was needed to cover a satellite station whose ambulance had left its base to respond to an emergency call. As we were getting close to the actual area the other ambulance vacated, we received a call for assistance in that same area.

There was a report of a man in his late twenties or early thirties running wild through the streets of a local tourist driven beach town. Nate and I lightly chuckled at what in our minds' eye that must have looked like. So in a non-emergency status we proceeded to drive to the middle of the small downtown area to where the police had a male subject in custody.

It seemed that the local city police received a call from a Greyhound passenger bus and were notified that a man was repeatedly committing disorderly conduct by continually yelling out to the bus driver to stop the bus. Unable to control the passenger, the bus driver had had enough and they were stopping at the next bus station to have the man removed. The police were now just awaiting our arrival for an evaluation of the person being detained and for the possible transportation of that person to a medical facility.

Upon our arrival, we noticed that at least two of the officers looked winded and a little disheveled from the chase that ensued after attempting to put the man that ran afoul on the bus into custody. As I exited the ambulance, I quickly looked over the man just to see whether he needed any immediate first-aid. He appeared at first glance to be physically unhurt.

I walked past the man who would momentarily become our patient, and approached the lead police officer. I asked what was going on and how can we be of assistance? The police officer told us that they had been chasing this guy for the better part of twenty minutes under and around several stopped buses, adjoining streets and alleys.

The officer said to me, "He surrendered to us about fifteen minutes ago and we're just waiting for you men to get here and take care of this guy."

"Has he given you any trouble or has been violent since being cuffed?" I asked.

"No, he's been fine and he's calmed down quite a bit."

"Okay, if you don't mind, I'll talk to him and see what his problem is and what he's trying to accomplish today. Has he said anything about what he's doing or where he's trying to get to?"

The officer said, "Yeah, he says he lives in Montreal, Canada and he's coming from Lake Charles, Louisiana, to see his kid and the kid's mother. Apparently, he is French Canadian and his English is really hard to understand."

I nodded in acknowledgement and approached our patient and introduced Nate and myself. I asked him his name. He hesitated for a moment, and then quickly stated his name.

I said to him, "Okay Alphonse, where are you from?"

He told me he was from Montreal and when I asked to see a driver's license or ID card one of the police officers at our patient's side quickly produced it and it did confirm his place of residence. When I asked his reason for going to Montreal, it was consistent with what he had previously stated to the police officers.

It was of no interest to me why or whether he was going to see his family or for that matter in which direction he was traveling. My only reason for asking him any social questions at all was merely to assess his mental cognition.

I asked him, "So, why are you in handcuffs right now?"

"I don't know. They (the police) were chasing me and when they caught me they put me in handcuffs and here I am."

"So you weren't being a problem on the bus."

"No."

"You weren't repeatedly yelling at the bus driver demanding he stop the bus?"

"Well, yeah, I was doing that."

"Why?"

"Because I was trying to get away from them!"

"Who is 'them' Alphonse?"

At the snap of a finger his eyes blazed with panic and he blurted out, "The people on the bus! They were trying to kill me!"

"Well they are gone and nobody here is trying to hurt you in any way, let alone kill you. Nate and I are here to help you. So are the police officers. They don't want you to get hurt; nor do they want you to accidentally hurt someone either. That's the only reason they had to stop you, Alphonse. The police and Nate and I just want everybody to be safe and secure. Do you understand that?"

"Yes," he replied as he looked down.

"Alphonse, don't look down. Look at me. Do you understand what I'm telling you? No one here is going to hurt you in any way. We are all here to help you and to get you to where you want to go. Do you understand that?"

After I sternly reassured Alphonse that we were all here to help him, I could see that the intensity in his eyes and the fear in his voice were subsiding as he looked right at me and said, "Yes, I understand what you are saying."

"Good, I'm glad to hear it. If I can get the officers to take those cuffs off of you, are you going to behave yourself?"

"Yes"

"Okay, because we don't want any trouble out of you. That's the deal. You don't give us any trouble and we will take you in the direction you were heading."

"What do you mean? By going in what direction?" he said in a startled voice.

I was immediately struck by how suddenly it was for our patient's anxiety to spike with the slightest bit of uncertainty on his part.

"Take it easy. Take it easy. Nate and I are paramedics with the ambulance here," as I gesture by raising my hand and pointing toward the ambulance. "We can only take you to a hospital. That's what we have to do. Now we can take you to the closest hospital, which is only eight or so miles away, but that puts you back in Indiana and further away from Montreal. Or we can take you almost thirty miles the other way to a different hospital, and get you that much closer to where your family lives?"

"Let's do that," he said as he started to fidget with the handcuffs.

"Okay, relax. We're going to get those cuffs off right now. Remember, I want no trouble and I mean no trouble at all, out of you."

As I'm giving Alphonse those instructions, a police officer removed his handcuffs. I told Nate to take Alphonse to the ambulance and get a set of vital signs. As I left Nate with Alphonse, I watched them walk to the ambulance, just to make sure that Alphonse didn't try to turn and run from us. As Nate ushered Alphonse into the patient compartment, and closed the door behind them, I turned to the lead officer. I told him that we were dealing with a patient who unquestionably has a real and genuine mental illness, and he wasn't just some guy having a bad day. We would be leaving momentarily to get him to our appropriate hospital of choice.

During the treatment and possible involuntary admittance of a psychiatric patient to a hospital, there are legal hurdles that have to be cleared. Those hurdles are high, and they should be. After all, it should be reasonably difficult to put someone behind lock and key for what someone else subjectively may think is a mental illness. Even so, I had little doubt that our patient would find himself in a mental ward by nightfall. I didn't want to further complicate the issue by taking our patient across a state line. The officer in charge acknowledged my rationale and I left him to attend to our patient and assist Nate.

As I opened the side door of the patient compartment of the ambulance, Nate had just completed recording the patient's vital signs, was fastening the lap belt around Alphonse and stated to me that he was ready to begin our trip.

The seat belt clicked together, and Alphonse looked up at Nate. Instantly, Nate said to him, "That's just a regular seat belt. Everyone who is a patient has to wear it if they are not lying on our cot."

Alphonse appeared to be satisfied with what Nate told him. I shut the door and walked over to the driver's side door, got behind the wheel and we were off to the hospital. For people who are not physically injured or ill, but are suffering from an alleged psychosis, the only thing that we are able to do is to transport them from point A to point B. We don't start IVs, we don't put people on our cardiac monitor, and we don't even restrain people unless they are violent. If EMS has a patient who is delusional, or believes his/her life is in danger, you attempt to restrain that patient by having them lay down on your ambulance cot. However, if you use restraining straps to hold them in place, you may be in for a real, and heated fight.

It's been my experience to be very low key with a patient who appears psychotic. Initiating small talk, thereby making them think about topics like the changing weather, how they are feeling and if they are comfortable are ways of redirecting a troubled mind in the early minutes of patient contact. You try to avoid making too much direct eye contact and you try to speak calmly, never raising your voice, being firm but understanding to their problems or challenges.

As an EMS provider, I don't want my patient to feel threatened in any way. Those patients with a mental disorder that would cause them to have irrational fears are particularly vulnerable. They have to be made to believe and understand that while they are in my ambulance they will be safe and I want them to believe that I am a friend who will be there to protect them and to help them.

From the driver's seat I could hear Nate talking calmly to Alphonse and saying that he would soon be at the hospital where he could get the help that he wanted and needed. I could hear him telling Alphonse that he had come a long way and he had to go just a little further to obtain his much needed treatment and medicine.

It's also been my experience that sometimes it just doesn't matter what is said to a patient struggling with reality. As we sped away, things went well for the first half of our trip. But as we continued, our patient became more concerned about where he was going. He asked questions such as: "Where are we going again? What's there? What am I going to do there? and Who's going to be there?"

Nate did his best to answer Alphonse's concerns as truthfully and in a manner to address his patient's growing doubts and suspicions. As all of this is going on, I'm rocketing the ambulance down the four-lane interstate highway in an effort to get Alphonse to the hospital as quickly as possible. During this particular trip I'm watching through the rearview mirror the interactions between my partner and our patient in the back of the ambulance more than the road ahead of me.

At about the twenty-four mile mark of our thirty-mile trek, the patient insisted that he now needed to look out of the back and side door windows of our ambulance. In order to do this, he needed to move around freely. Nate did his best in trying to explain to an ever more fearful, argumentative, and agitated patient that everything was going to be all right, and that for his safety he had to remain seated with his lap belt in place.

It was no use. It was becoming increasingly difficult for Nate to keep his patient quiet and sitting still. Every time Nate would say, "C'mon Alphonse, you have to remain seated and belted in," Alphonse would wait ten to fifteen seconds and release himself from his lap belt and get to one of the windows on each of the three doors.

Each time Nate would tell his patient that, "everything was going to be alright and that I'm here just to help you," the more untrusting and afraid he became. It was now becoming harder for Nate to handle Alphonse, as he was constantly releasing his belt in attempt to get to one of the windowed doors.

Finally after watching this for the last five or so minutes, I yelled back to my partner, "Nate, keep him down! Or do you need me to come back there?"

"No. I got him." Nate replied.

Sensing that he was starting to lose control of his patient, Nate really got into his face about sitting still. It is vital that any patient and particularly a possible psychotic one needs to be physically secured in the patient compartment of the ambulance. This is for their protection as well as for the security of the attending EMS provider. It seemed to work well for the next two or three minutes.

As we are flying down the interstate highway at eighty-five miles per hour, I made known our intention of leaving the highway by turning on the right turn signal. I began to ramp-off at our designated exit point. At that moment, I took my attention away from the back of the ambulance, and concentrated on the braking and slowing down.

As soon as I had taken my concern away from the activities behind me, and put them toward not running off of the exit ramp, I heard Nate yell out, "HEY!" I snapped my eyes to the rearview mirror. I saw the patient was again, at the back double doors of the ambulance attempting to open one of them. Because he was trying to escape, I knew that Nate and I would have to physically take down and restrain Alphonse.

In an attempt to knock him off of his feet, I hit the brakes as hard and as fast as I could. Usually this is done because the EMS staff member attending to the patient is in a fight or some kind of physical altercation. On this particular day it was done in an attempt to prevent Alphonse's escape from our protection and care. Even so, I knew that as soon as I got the ambulance stopped, Nate and I were going to be in for a fight.

While I was standing on the brakes with both feet, I was simultaneously reaching for the ambulance communications radio and telling our dispatcher that we needed help from law enforcement immediately at Exit 22 on the U.S. 31 bypass. As all of this is taking place, I didn't feel the sudden lurch of the vehicle that I expected when hitting the brakes so suddenly.

Instead, it felt as though I was driving over a rumble strip or a giant washboard and the ambulance was decelerating at a much slower rate. This was because the ambulance was outfitted with an anti-lock brake system. That system does not allow for the near abrupt stop that skidding to a stop on dry pavement would allow. The result was that I could see that I didn't send the patient reeling as anticipated, and so the patient remained at the back doors. Worse yet, Nate was having trouble getting to him.

In a matter of just five seconds, I had the ambulance stopped, had my seat belt unbuckled, slammed the ambulance into park and was bolting out of the driver's door and toward the back of the ambulance. During that time, Nate had made his way to the patient and attempted to hold him until I got there. In this short amount of time the patient had gotten the back door open, slithered out of his heavy coat that he was wearing and escaped Nate's grip as well as the confines of the back of the ambulance.

I couldn't believe what had just happened. In a matter of two seconds from when I left the driver's door and until I reached the back of the ambulance, the patient was already more than fifty feet from us. I gave a brief chase until be abruptly turned toward the shoulder of the highway and leaped over the barrier fence and into the darkness.

"I can't believe it!" I screamed. "Come on Nate, we've got to find this guy!"

We raced back to the ambulance and hurriedly drove around to where we thought he might be heading. Once in the ambulance, Nate told me that he couldn't believe how fast he was able to shed his coat and escape. Although I didn't say it at the time, I was disappointed that once I got the ambulance stopped, my partner was unable to hold our patient for at least two seconds. In a way, I was angry with Nate, but not nearly as much as I was with the man we were there to help.

I tried to keep in mind, that he was legitimately sick and was simply attempting to escape some imagined threat. All of the patience, understanding, consoling and encouragement Nate put forth to Alphonse; the unending effort to keep him quiet, calm and secure and doing it over and over again was now all for naught. Now, I just wanted to grab this guy and throw him back into the ambulance and tie him to the stretcher.

When Nate and I last saw Alphonse, he was running across a large, open field filled with tall weeds, toward the general direction of a large industrial park. Once there, I thought he would be very difficult to find and harder yet to detain. To our surprise and relief, Nate and I spotted Alphonse standing out in the open talking to three employees of a local fruit cannery depot. I didn't take the time to maneuver around the driveways. Instead, I drove the ambulance across several small yards, sidewalks and parking lot islands and stopped the ambulance to within thirty feet of him. Nate and I jumped out of the rig and immediately started briskly walking toward our patient.

"Hey man, you can't do this!" I yelled, "You can't just jump out of our ambulance and run off like that!"

Not thinking that my actions might cause his level of fear and trepidation to markedly increase, he suddenly turns and sprints away from us. Nate and I at once started to chase Alphonse in an attempt to capture him. From that point forward there was no more talking. The only sounds are feet hitting asphalt and those of quick and then heavy and finally exhausted breathing. I ran as fast as I could, and I was slowly catching up to him to the point to where I was able to touch the back of his shirt.

Although I was within as little as two inches from getting a firm grasp on our fleeing and elusive runner, it would be the closest I would ever get to him again. Within the span of about fifteen seconds, and at least a hundred yards later, I was out of breath. We were running in tall weeds, and our object of pursuit had vanished into the darkness.

Once again, he was gone. Coming so close and not being able to catch and detain Alphonse in order to get him the help he so desperately needed was acutely frustrating and left me as aggravated as I could be.

Without our flashlights or personal radio equipment, Nate and I had no chance of finding him. As a result and still trying to catch our breath, Nate and I turned away from the black abyss Alphonse had entered and jogged back to where our ambulance was parked. We conveyed to our dispatch center what had just transpired and started to look once again for a frightened and perhaps terrified individual.

Within a minute or two our supervisor, Mike Schultz, who was heading our way after our first call for help was on scene. I told Nate to go with Mike and keep looking as well as brief him on what had happened and how we ended up in this escalating fiasco.

Shortly after Nate joined Mike in the search for Alphonse, Michigan State Trooper (MSP), Bernum arrived in her squad car and said, "Jim, what happened?"

Without trying to hide my disgust I replied, "This clown jumped out of our ambulance as we were exiting the highway! We found him and we almost caught up with him, but he eluded us again."

"You've got to be kidding. He just jumped out of the ambulance?"

"Yeah, that's what happened. Listen Melissa, with all of the residential subdivisions around here," gesturing with my hand in one direction and then another, "he's obviously not armed, but he should definitely be considered dangerous. This guy is truly psychotic."

She nodded and sped off to start to look for our elusive patient and I quickly returned to my ambulance to do the same. Once inside the ambulance I used the bright, twin load lights that are on both side and the rear of the box of the ambulance to illuminate a general area around the ambulance for a distance of about twenty yards. I used our unit's spotlight to look further into the darkness.

I drove around for several minutes hoping to find some sign of Alphonse. This particular industrial park had many businesses, scores of warehouses, garages and various outbuildings that are both lit and those that are dark, stacks of wood pallets, heavy trucks and other equipment. It eventually became necessary for me get out of the ambulance and search on foot. I walked through and around all of it with a flashlight in one hand, and a walkie-talkie in the other. Although I wasn't absolutely sure, I wasn't too concerned about being surprised or ambushed by Alphonse. I was relatively confident that the "fight or flight" response that happens to any human when scared or frightened would in this case result in flight. In essence I wasn't afraid of being attacked while walking around by myself in the dark, looking for a deeply psychotic individual.

After being on foot for perhaps twenty minutes and not seeing a hint of someone lurking about, I walked back to the ambulance. Within a few seconds of reaching the ambulance, our crew chief dropped off Nate so he and I could continue the search. By this time there were many squad cars from several police agencies searching for our missing man. The three of us briefly discussed where Alphonse might be hiding or lurking about.

We concluded that since no one from law enforcement or EMS has spotted him, he could very well be more than a mile from where we last saw him. He could be in somebody's home, doing God knows what. He could have double backed toward the interstate highway or he could be within fifty feet from where Mike, Nate and I were standing, hiding in the tall weeds or a shadowy corner of the cannery or another warehouse. In short, we had no idea of where to look. We needed to continue our quest, but it was becoming more and more apparent that he was gone.

At least that's what I thought.

Mike drove away in his crew chief vehicle and Nate and I were just discussing where to look next when all of a sudden our dispatch radio that had been relatively quiet suddenly came alive with the Berrien County Sheriff Department's dispatcher calling out to Medic's dispatcher, Brandi. "Go ahead with your traffic Berrien." she replied.

"Medic, we have a report of a pedestrian P.I. (personal injury accident) at the 22-Mile marker on the U.S. 31 bypass."

"Clear on it Berrien. Break, 40-10 (our ambulance call sign) are you clear on Berrien's traffic?"

With some nervousness and certain resignation, I confirmed to Brandi that I did indeed hear what Berrien stated. Instantly, I knew without a doubt, that Alphonse had been struck by a motor vehicle of some kind. Perhaps with a lot of luck, he wouldn't be hurt too badly. I quickly flipped our emergency lights on, as Nate and I sped to where the county sheriff dispatcher said our new, and possibly old patient, was located.

Actually, nobody knew for sure whether the person who had been struck on the highway was the same person who had escaped from Nate and me forty minutes earlier, but what was the chance it wasn't? For me it was zero.

When we were perhaps just a minute away, Brandi came back over the radio and said, "Dispatch to 40-10." I grabbed the mike and said, "Go ahead Brandi."

"MSP is on scene at the 22 and says the MVA victim is a K."

My heart sunk with that news. What Brandi said was that the Michigan State Police had located our patient at the 22-Mile marker on the U.S. 31 bypass and had been killed by being struck by a motor vehicle. I looked over to Nate. I thought he was going to be sick.

As we rolled up to where the squad cars had parked on the shoulder of the median strip, we both saw the body laying on the grassy edge of the pavement. As I exited the ambulance, my good friend and MSP trooper Jim Janes had told me that a young twenty-three-year old driver of a car and his twenty-year-old girlfriend had stopped after the sudden impact. They told trooper Janes that they thought that they had unexpectedly hit a deer. Apparently it was that fast. The young couple stated that there was no warning and that neither of them had seen the man run out in front of them until a split second before the unforeseen impact.

Nate and I approached the body to further examine and to confirm his death. It was obvious from his head injuries alone that he was killed on impact and died instantly. We also established with certainty that it was indeed the deeply psychotic person that had escaped from us earlier. Nate looked to me perhaps to say something or to see what we are supposed to do next. I looked at one of the nicest guys to ever work at Medic and it was easy to see just how bad he felt about this whole sorry episode.

I told him, "Hey Nate, we did the best that we could. There wasn't a thing you did or didn't do in the back of the ambulance that I would have done or not done. So don't beat yourself up about this. It's okay to feel bad, because this poor guy was legitimately, mentally sick. There's no doubt about that either. And I'm going to tell you something else; don't let anyone at Medic give you any grief about this, and that means supervisors too. They may want to joke and tease you about it, but it's not a damn bit funny. This was a tragedy in every sense of the word. So if anybody and I mean anybody wants to second-guess you; just tell them to kiss your ass! "

Nate tried to chuckle a little bit about my last comment. But it's true. This was a tragedy that through a devastating mental illness, a young man lost his life. I'll never be able to fathom what must have gone through the last few minutes of this tortured man's mind. Because of that, it was impossible for me to fully appreciate the extent of Alphonse's psychosis, and just how he was on the "razor's edge" of losing any modicum of self-control or civil behavior.

I didn't realize that his inability for restraint would easily and quickly evaporate into irrational thought and subsequent actions. My supposition is that Alphonse's paranoia rapidly became a frantic necessity to break away from the limitations and restrictions of the patient compartment of an ambulance. Therefore, I think that at all costs, he needed to run.

And without having any substantive history with Alphonse, I sense he ran countless times from only God knows how many imagined threats long before Nate and I ever came into contact with him. In the end and during the last moments of this anguished man's life, I believe he had to run from the all too familiar pain of a primal fear incarcerated in a tormented mind from which there was no escape.

EPILOGUE

You've just read a small sampling of a career in EMS, that is the real deal. It's a long life in EMS that spans more than thirty-five years in time, and encompasses in the neighborhood of 30,000 or more ambulance calls. After that lengthy amount of time and that many calls for help and assistance, I firmly believe that there isn't a medical illness or traumatic injury scenario that I haven't seen or haven't been involved with.

Whether you are currently a Medical First Responder, an EMT, a Paramedic—volunteer or professional—you will have found a certain camaraderie within these pages. Some of it may have reminded you of fond, as well as unpleasant memories. Some of it may have made you laugh out loud, as you may have your own "Aggie and Herbie" to deal with. Some of it may have torn open an emotional scab that you wished was left alone.

If you are contemplating such a career or involvement, some of the preceding pages are a cross section look at society, complete with all of its thrills and ills as seen through the eyes of a longtime EMS provider. If you choose a career in EMS, most of it can be a reasonable expectation.

If you are already an EMS provider, I'm sure you've witnessed many things in your career that you can identify with in this writing. If you have worked regularly for several years in EMS, you already know what it's like to be on the front lines, battling morbidity as well as mortality. You know what it's like to see people of every stripe and color at their worst, while you attempt to perform at your very best. Because of that, you already know it's pretty much a thankless job.

But, you also have to know and must never forget that what you do is vital to your community. EMS promotes and enhances a greater quality of life to those communities that are well served by highly trained and educated people who are dedicated to the pre-hospital phase of emergency healthcare. Therefore a cogent argument can be made that EMS is every bit as essential to a high quality of life to the citizens of any community as any police or fire department.

Oddly enough, you'll find out and might even be dismayed over the fact that seldom will you get that pat on the back that you deserve and may need for a tough job done well. You may never or all too infrequently get that thank you for relieving pain and suffering, giving emergency aid and providing comfort.

But know this: you are doing the Lord's work. You are helping your fellow man. By relieving the agony of pain from illness and injury, you are agents of goodness. Be content with that.

COMMENTARY
Banging My Head Against The Wall

What would a book on the subject of a life in EMS be without saying a few things regarding the politically charged systemic problems that have become serious if not critical in the health care delivery structure? Think of that structure as a bicycle wheel. The center of that wheel is "the health care problem." Each of the spokes of the wheel represents a serious problem in medicine and all the many spokes represent the wheel of a very complex industry. There are probably a dozen or more issues (spokes) that lead directly or indirectly to the health care problem.

As evidenced, you can't turn on the six o'clock news, open a newspaper or listen to a radio without hearing some political pundit talking about this or that, without them spouting off about the exorbitant and ever-escalating cost of health care in this country. They extol the fact of obscene profits made by the big drug companies. They demonize those companies for what they see as an unreasonable charge or cost to the public. They seem to conveniently forget that the public depends on those same pharmaceutical companies to produce the next generation of drugs to fight countless diseases and maladies. The cost in time and money for the research and development of medicines are measured by decades and hundreds of millions of dollars.

Personally speaking, I have two sons. Both of them have been afflicted with Type 1 (juvenile onset) diabetes. What has happened is that each of their immune systems (the system that fights disease and infection) has targeted as a foreign body and subsequently destroyed the part of their pancreas that produces insulin.

What that means personally as well as medically for each of my sons now is that in order to live they need to take insulin several times a day via a syringe and needle or insulin pump. They must always check their blood glucose (sugar) levels in their blood an average of four times a day. The two of them must see from time to time a medical doctor who specializes in endocrinology. They also see a retinologist to care for their eyesight. They must always make sure that they care for even the most superficial cuts and scrapes. Catching the ordinary flu can and has landed them in the hospital.

My sons are well aware of the long-term effects of this insidious disease. They know of the blindness caused by retinopathy, kidney disease and failure (nephropathy), heart disease (cardiomyopathy), limb amputation (neuropathy). All of these diseases are the direct cause of not being able to adequately control the exact amount of glucose in your blood stream at any given time.

Each of our pancreases is able to produce the exact amount of insulin that our bodies need for metabolizing our food intake. When your pancreas is unable to continue to create this naturally occurring life-sustaining hormone, you have to take injections of synthetically produced insulin just to survive. The trouble is that it can be incredibly difficult to regulate artificially what the body does naturally. The result of a poorly controlled blood glucose level is all too often the realization of the aforementioned diseases. So you'll have to excuse me if I don't seem to have a big problem with the drug companies making enough money to hire the best and the brightest of bioresearch scientists to someday find a cure for my two sons and millions of sons and daughters just like them.

To continue, the pundits also wring their white-knuckled hands over the costs to see a doctor who is a specialist in this area or that area of medicine. Never mind that the "medical specialist" (depending on their specialty) may have spent up to a dozen years or more in didactic and clinical training and many hundreds of thousands of dollars obtaining the needed education and schooling.

Of course, the biggest "bad guy" of the bunch seems to be those nasty and uncaring health insurance companies. Whether it is Medicare, Medicaid, BXBS or any other of the HMO's or PPO's, I always seem to hear how "they just don't care." And the biggest one lately seems to be the cost of that "just gotta have it" wonder medicine.

There are for sure many problems that include but are probably not limited to not only what I just mentioned above but also the American Medical Association's reluctance to do a better job in weeding out incompetent or ineffective doctors. The high cost of litigation with what I believe to be more times than not, obscene legal and lawyer fees. Confiscatory malpractice insurance premiums and useless and redundant medical tests, all lend to ever-escalating costs to every citizen and business in this country.

The previous four items listed are inexorably linked. If the wizards of smart that we call Federal as well as State politicians want to do something productive, they should deal with each of those four problems as one big intertwined problem. It should be recognized that unless each of those four problems are dealt with simultaneously, just as broken spokes of a bicycle wheel need to be fixed, some of the biggest problems will have no chance of being solved.

Like any other massive and nationwide business or industry, there is probably a fair amount of greed, corruption and outright fraud. All of that may very well be true, but I, for one, can't speak to any of them from a totally informed point of view.

Yes, I've heard over the years, several different doctors talk about malpractice costs and how it affects their bottom line. At the same time, I have personally witnessed incompetent doctors practicing medicine in more than one emergency room and I know of pharmacists who have called doctors to clarify a prescription for the correct medicine, dosage and duration. I have also seen nurses and more than a few paramedics who weren't, shall we say, right for the job.

Like any other field of endeavor, there's a chance that medicine may not be for just anyone. So let us say for sure that there are several problems with the delivery as well as the funding of health care in this country.

Who pays? Is it a right or a requirement to receive needed health care? Is it neither? Is it a personal responsibility to fund your own family's health care or a corporate obligation? Is it the duty of the Federal or State government to fund health care for those who are senior citizens and those who are legitimately disabled? Should it be the unwavering commitment of those governments to entitle national health care to each and every legal (and most likely illegal) resident of this country?

If there's anything that's a problem in this country, it's usually because there is a dollar sign attached to it. Medicine is certainly no different. According to Kaiser Health News, total medical costs in the United States in 2008 eclipsed 2.3 trillion dollars. That's more than three times as high as it was in just 1990 (714 billion dollars).

Medically speaking and from A to Z, $7,681 was spent on each and every American. That astronomical sum of treasure is 16.2% of our nation's Gross Domestic Product (GDP). That means that for every $100 spent for goods and services (that takes into account food, housing, clothing, education, entertainment, transportation, infra-structure, taxes at every level and a thousand other things), $16.20 was spent on everything from Band-Aids to multi-organ transplants. In other words, for every six dollars plunked down to pay for something, more than one of those dollars was snatched up for health care costs.

Forbes Magazine reported in 2013, the total health care cost shot up to 3.6 trillion. The increase continued in 2014, reaching 3.8 trillion and is expected to hit the four trillion mark in 2015. If the post-war baby boomers retire at the age of 65, ten thousand will retire everyday for the next two decades. With the associated age-related diseases many senior citizens incur, the money that will have to be spent threatens to crush our economy.

The four parts of an intertwined problem that I listed earlier is from an observed opinion that for me forms a circular problem (bad docs, high litigation settlements, exorbitant legal fees and silly and or redundant medical tests). The part that I "know" a little bit about is the emergency health care side of things as I've been in the ambulance business since June 1977. I think that's a long time to get a feel for what is right and what is wrong with this small part of the medical industry as compared to the whole.

I can tell you one thing for certain; and that's the emergency health care system is broken. The emergency room, in part, has become little more than a dumping ground for private practicing doctors who can't or usually don't want to see their own patients for whatever reason.

It used to be that if you called your doctor because you had a per-sistent cough, a cold or the sniffles, that many times that doctor may just call in a prescription for this or for that to your local pharmacy. If you weren't feeling any better by the time you were finished with your prescribed medication, you made an appointment to see your doctor for follow-up care. Not anymore.

Now, for legal and not medical reasons, that's simply not the case. Nobody wants the liability of that truly one in a thousand times or maybe one in ten thousand cases where the prescribed medicine didn't do what was intended or somebody had some adverse outcome from the over the phone diagnosing. As a result, they just advise their patients to go to the local hospital's emergency room.

I'm not advocating that any doctor, regardless of their medical specialty, should try to diagnose and analyze cardiac chest pain or acute abdominal pain over the phone. What I'm saying is why can't the most common of minor maladies that each of us faces a few times per year be handled over the phone? Of course that's if you think you need to see your doctor for the first signs of a cold, cough or flu. Come on people, get real and suck it up!

You don't have to run to the nearest doctor's office, walk-in clinic or hospital emergency room after the first sneeze! However, we do because we have insurance that will pay for this trivial silliness. In the end this kind of thinking costs everyone a whole lot of money! Somehow the general public has forgotten what insurance is and how it is supposed to be used. It was never designed to be what it has now become, and that is as a third party payer for every nickel and dime thing that comes by.

Another thing insurance was never intended or designed to do was to pick up the cost of your medicines. Why is it that when we see a particular medicine advertised on TV advocating the ability to do this or that, we seem to know better than a medical doctor? Why is it that we think that we just have to have the latest drug on the market when perhaps a "tried and true" generic drug would be more than adequate?

It's because too many people think that since they have health insurance with a prescription card benefit that affords them a co-pay of pennies on a dollar, it doesn't matter. The true cost of that medicine is either ignored, not considered or isn't known by the consumer-patient in the first place. But make no mistake about it, the cost of that fancy designer drug is still there and somebody somewhere is paying for it. You can bet everybody's bottom line on that.

What insurance was originally designed to do was to pick up the high dollar cost of major events. Things like paying for the cost of treating heart disease, cancers, traumatic injury and the like. In other words, insurance was designed to keep you out of the poor house, not as an all-encompassing payer for every medical need.

The fall-out of the mind set that your insurance company must pay for literally seeing a doctor for the "sniffles" and the obligatory "feel good" prescription medicine is at least partially responsible if not fully responsible for the exploding health care costs in this country. If you are naïve enough to think that since you don't pay the actual up-front cost of this test or that drug, or that you don't pay for it at all; think again.

Another thing we all get to pay for is the insurance company's middlemen and the layer upon layer of complicated administration. Almost all of us have had to deal with "the voice on the other end of the phone" that tells you that the latest test or procedure that your medical doctor has ordered for your health care isn't covered by your particular health care plan. If it is covered, then they will explain why there is a deductible, co-pay or why only a percentage of the test or procedure is covered. Then when you get your Explanation Of Benefits (EOB) in the mail, it will invariably not match what you were told over the phone! The whole thing is sheer lunacy!

If you work for a company, corporation or organization that has employed sponsored health care as a benefit; it's paying or in the end will pay the lion's share of the cost of your medical needs. As a result, they must pass on those increased expenses of doing business to the consumers of this country in the form of higher costs for goods and services.

Further fall-out is that the local emergency rooms across any town or city in America have become inundated and over burdened with clinic patients on top of the true emergency patients they already see. What's worse yet is that a good share of the people who were told to go to the local emergency room by their doctor, in turn call 911 for an ambulance ride to that hospital. I can't begin to tell you how many of our ambulance calls are truly just really expensive taxi rides. I can tell you with all certainty that it is over one-half.

One of the unintended consequences of an all-encompassing medical payer is that there are problems getting them to pay for it all. Just about everybody that has inquired about minor out-patient surgery to those who have need of protracted in-patient treatment and long term care have had to deal with complicated and confusing paperwork. Numerous phone calls that involve being put on hold for several minutes at a time and switched from one bureaucrat to another and then another are evidence of a multi-layered insurance administrative system that is at times frustrating and exasperating.

Not too long ago and just one example out of thousands, Medic 1 transported an eighty-two- year-old lady to the local emergency room because she was advised by her doctor to go to the hospital to be treated for a blister on her forefinger. I kid you not! And do you know why? One big reason: medical liability and how it's precluded the use of good, old-fashioned, common sense.

I mean, if you think you just have to do something, what's wrong with putting a Band-Aid on it and protecting it? A Band-Aid probably costs about a dime. The cost of just the ambulance ride is more than $200 of taxpayer's money if your third party payer is Medicaid. If you have your own insurance plan or if you pay out of pocket, it will be far in excess of $700! I think that's just a little too much money to spend for a common ordinary blister that's on your finger.

All of that nonsense is solely because of the fear of medical liability and civil litigation. Good doctors who own their own practices, or are in a partnership with a group of like-minded medical practitioners that share the same specialty, fear the fall-out of possibly losing their practices. If those same doctors are contracted with a hospital emergency department, they fear the loss of their jobs.

To continue, let us not forget that the $200- $700 cost is just the cost of having someone like myself come to your house or wherever you may be currently staying to rescue you from your dreaded blister. I, or any one of my many colleagues, will be there to give you an ordinary everyday ride to the hospital. It's the same ride that you could have and should have gotten on your own. It's the same ride that should never be the obligation of EMS.

To continue this absurdity, once you're at the hospital, there will be an emergency room charge and the doctor will have a charge for you as well. More than likely the doctor will charge you a fee to say, "You've got a blister. Keep it covered for a few days and you'll be fine."

I'm sure each hospital and its doctor groups are different, but I wouldn't be surprised at all, if the hospital charges didn't far exceed the ambulance fees. And God help you if you have a pre-existing medical problem that is chronic in nature. Let's just say for instance, that you have a long history of a lung disease, and you need oxygen once in a while. Even though you are not short of breath now, you don't need oxygen now, and your blister has nothing at all with your chronic lung disease, watch out. Because, here comes the blood tests, blood gases, chest x-rays, and probably the routine EKG. Before you know it, "somebody"—whether it is you or an insurance company—has a $2,000-$3,000 bill coming your (or their) way.

The point is this, if that person were personally responsible for the costs incurred, there would be a ninety-nine percent chance the lady with a blister would forego her trip to the hospital altogether. The fact of the matter is that, as a result, we as the consumers of medical services rarely see (let alone are responsible for) the total cost of medical care. We as a society are not as concerned nearly as much as we should be for the actual charges incurred. Another truism, is that the more we expect and demand our health insurance companies to cover in medical fees and charges for this type of misuse and abuse, the higher our health insurance premiums become. It's economics 101. The old proverb that says, that there is "no such thing as a free lunch," couldn't be more valid.

What about the working poor who struggle to put food on the table and keep a roof over their children's heads? More often than not, they don't have private or job-related benefits that would afford them health care. Too many don't have Medicaid and therefore don't seek medical attention and appropriate treatment when it is warranted. If the lady with the blister on her finger had to pay out of her own pocket for all of the treatment that was afforded her for such foolishness, just think of the money that would be saved or better spent on the truly needy in our society.

Let's continue our honesty for just a moment. Another reason the good doctor who told the lady to seek medical attention at the local emergency room (even though this type of care is the most expensive way to receive any kind of care) is because of intellectual laziness. Rather than talking to the patient in question, or talking with the patient's responsible health care advocate, it's just "easier" for the doctor to totally absolve him/herself from any and all responsibility and liability. By doing this, they push off this type of expensive silliness onto an already overloaded hospital emergency room system.

Once at the local hospital emergency room, there will be the usual routine medical tests that have little to nothing to do with the perceived problem at hand. The number one reason for these tests has nothing to do with the problem at hand. It is…you guessed it, the fear of civil liability and litigation. That fear is pervasive, palpable and it is without a doubt what drives the absurd tests that are routinely performed on a person with a blister on their forefinger. Consequently, it drives the overall price tag as well.

Let me give you another generic example.

Many, many times over the years I've had a twenty-something or a thirty-something year old male who will call or have someone call an ambulance for him. It will eventually come out that this person twisted his ankle playing a pickup game of basketball. Typically this patient limped home or was driven to his home and then called EMS for "a ride" to the hospital. Invariably, this patient will have Medicaid and sometimes Medicare.

After checking his injury, I'll say, "You have a sprain. Put some ice on it and stay off of it for a day or two."

Then he'll tell me that he wants to go to the hospital. I'll look at him and say, "Well, go to the hospital."

He responds by saying, "I want you to take me."

I already knew that but I'll look back at him and say, "You mean you want me to take you to the hospital by ambulance for a minor ankle sprain?"

He will respond by saying, "Yeah, what's wrong with that?"

…Now, I have to tell him, 'what's wrong with that'.

"Well, first off, most men I know wouldn't call an ambulance for a sprained ankle. Secondly, do you have insurance through your place of employment?" I'm fairly certain I already know the answer so it's a rhetorical question.

"No man, I don't work. I'm on disability," he'll say.

Asking him further, "What do you mean you're on disability? What's your disability?" Almost invariably the answer is he has a history of seizures, has a "bad back" or headaches.

So, whichever of the usual three he answers me with I'll say back to him, "Oh I see, you aren't healthy enough to earn a living, but your healthy enough to play a physical game of basketball and hurt yourself doing that? So, tell me, who is the quack doctor you saw who said that at the age of (whatever), you can't work for the rest of your life? Who was it that said that you're going to grow old and all the while you're going to be nothing more than a drag on society? Who said that to you? That's a terrible thing to say to a young man!"

Usually by this time by the look on his face and from my perspective, the patient is more often than not really pissed off with me. I guess I can't blame him. After all, I've called into question his manhood, his societal usefulness and his more than willingness to sit on his ass and collect a welfare check for the remainder of his entire life.

As I continue, I will say something to the effect of, "Well if you still want to go to the emergency room, and since you limped into the house, you can limp out to the ambulance, because the last thing I'm going to do is carry you. But don't worry; the working taxpayers will be more than happy to give you your free ride to the hospital. Don't forget to bring your Master-caid (Medicaid) card with you. I'll need to get the numbers off of it. And by the way, since you could have found your own way to the hospital and this is as far as it gets from life or limb threatening, Medicaid probably will not pay the bill. That will make you totally responsible for the payment in full. Just so you know you'll have to sign your name to a statement that says you understand and agree to that."

Well, sometimes it works and the social delinquent stays home and takes care of himself. As far as I'm concerned, that's scoring one for the working, tax paying public. Like I said, that's "sometimes". What usually happens in this particular generic incident is that he ends up limping out to the ambulance where I record his vital signs. He then signs his name to the statement that I just explained to him. He and I both know he still has no intention of paying for the EMS services provided to him and that his signature means little to nothing. At that point my partner and I will drive him to the local hospital and dump him at the triage department.

Once there, a registered nurse will see him. That nurse will call that patient into a small exam room and record the patient's medical history, find out the particulars about the injury, record another set of vital signs and finally he will be told to take a seat and wait his turn for non-emergency status patients.

As this generic patient waits and waits and waits to be seen, often he will get tired of waiting and will call somebody on his cell phone. He'll then get up and leave the hospital before ever being seen by the attending emergency room physician. This is the same guy who was hurt so badly that he needed EMS to attend to him for his injury. Finally, within a few minutes, a friend will be there to pick him up from the emergency room and he will leave; the same friend he couldn't call to give him a ride to a local walk-in clinic.

Some people think that I might be a little over the top with this evaluation. I'll give you that. I might be. But honestly speaking, I'm okay with it. It's just that I really despise people who misuse and abuse EMS for convenience and for merely a taxi ride and especially if they make a habit of calling us for their "free ride". Sometimes I argue with them. Sometimes I just say, "Get in the ambulance and let's go." More than not, it just depends on my mood at the time.

It matters whether or not I've been running my ass off for nearly eighteen straight hours with very little time off in between calls. It matters if I've had real, true emergencies that day or not. It matters whether I've been thinking about how much time I spend working to support my family. Finally, it matters whether they truly don't know any better or if they have that "you owe me" mentality.

On occasion that same guy with the ankle sprain will call back an hour later from his home and demand that EMS take him back again to the hospital? Again, I kid you not! Believe me when I tell you, it happens! It's an outrageous abuse of the system that costs the taxpayer huge sums of money. That's resources that are becoming scarcer every day.

It's also the reason insured patients pay a minimum of $700 for ambulance transportation rather than the $200 bill afforded government sponsored insurance recipients or for those people that have no insurance and have no intention of paying for the use (or misuse) of the local EMS service. The productive tax-payer gets it from both ends; higher taxes for what amounts to insufficient government reimbursements and is presented privately with a much more costly bill, for the singular reason of having to subsidize those same inadequate reimbursements.

I can't begin to tell you about the hundreds of times that I've taken the pregnant teenager to the obstetrical unit at the hospital who has just started her labor and more often than not whose labor pains are ten to fifteen minutes apart. The chances of a delivery of that baby in that scenario in the five to fifteen minutes that I'll be with the expectant mother, traveling at the rate of normal traffic speed, (no lights or sirens type of ride to the hospital) is probably about zero.

Yet right behind the ambulance will be a car loaded with Mom, the siblings, best friends, and whoever else. Just as easily, she too could (and of course should) be riding to the hospital in that same car. But no, for some reason, we need the high tech, highly-trained staff and equipment of EMS to give what otherwise is just a really expensive taxi ride to the hospital.

I truly don't know if it's a lack of common sense, a sense of entitlement, or the fact that there is no co-pay or monetary charge of any kind. However, I do know this. If I were able to say to that particular person that I absolutely know without a doubt who could and certainly should go by private vehicle to the hospital (that is if they thought they needed to go at all); that I don't want to hear about co-pays or deductibles for services or any hard luck story. It would cost them $5 out of their own pocket before they could get into the patient compartment of my ambulance, they wouldn't go. They'd just stay home or they would find their own way.

Think about that. They'll think absolutely nothing of incurring a charge to the taxpaying public of a minimum of $200 or perhaps a charge in excess of $700 to a private third party payer. But if I as an EMS provider could say that this ride would cost them, out of pocket, just $5, there is positively no doubt in my mind, that they would not use the ambulance. In my mind, this is nothing less than an everyday example of a parasitic pathology demonstrated at the human level through thought and action.

As angry and as pissed off as I get, I know that I'm just "beating my head against the wall." I know that there is no possible way for me to change this type of abuse and misuse of the EMS system. I know that untold millions and most likely billions of dollars are just wasted away in this everyday way of life in EMS. Worse yet is that I know that in the big picture, this is just a "drop in the bucket".

What do you or what can you say when you look at somebody's list of medicine and see amongst this or that a bottle of prescription filled 81mg. (baby) aspirin. I think that little thing, is the one thing that just infuriates me the most. Think of it. There are people out there who would rather soak the taxpayer for aspirin that you could buy yourself in generic bulk form at a rate of a hundred or more aspirin for two dollars! What do you say to that person who won't even buy over the counter generic aspirin for themselves? They don't so much as blink an eye when they hand that nonsensical prescription to the local pharmacist.

And what about the dopey doctor that writes that idiotic prescription? He's not dopey. He's just afraid of the cost of litigation. That good doctor is afraid that unless he makes absolutely sure (by writing that prescription for 81mg. Aspirin) that his patient gets that aspirin, that unless it is "free", he won't buy it for himself.

Do you see now how "off the charts" we've become with this total lack of personal responsibility? Do you see now why medical costs are increasing annually much more than the rate of inflation? That's just a very small example of what I see everyday as a paramedic in the emergency health care end of medicine!

For me, it's a great indicator of a truly lazy, slothful and pathologic part of society. This pathological behavior has got to be curtailed. I believe that adults of every stripe react to two things: pain and money. Since I'm not advocating beating anybody into submission over their misuse of EMS and the emergency department at the local hospital, I guess I'm advocating that people who rely on the benevolence of the American tax-paying public be a whole lot more responsible for their decisions and actions.

I truly believe that co-pays although might not be the best or final answer, do have a place in the improvement of responsible behavior. If something such as that is instituted, then and only then will that person have a financially based, vested interest.

It's amazing how different people will act if they are at least in some small part spending their own money and not somebody else's money.

The most telling thing is this: I have an acquaintance who works for the local Department of Social Services. She tells me that she sees and tends to the needs of around 300 clients. Out of those 300, she tells me that an easy 75% are "scammers" and that the total could be as high as 90%. To say the least, when I queried her about this little known fact, I was stunned. My goodness, I knew the number might be high (50% or maybe a little more), but 75-90%? I find myself getting depressed if I think about it too long. When you see the scope of this abuse and misuse on a daily basis, it's really disheartening.

For me, the reason I find it so distressing and disheartening is because I know there are millions upon millions of senior citizens who need better health care and prescription drug cost relief. There are also millions of legitimately disabled Americans who depend on government-sponsored programs as well.

As a society, we should be doing a better job of screening and ascertaining who should be eligible for such taxpayer funded health care. A much more stringent and higher threshold of "disability" should be formulated and put into effect. Why should someone who is a chronic alcoholic or an illicit drug abuser be eligible for disability and therefore government sponsored Medicare health insurance? They aren't people with disabilities. They are people with weaknesses who live a lifestyle that is more often than not enabled by the well-meaning American public!

At some level, those people know that if they get intoxicated or stoned and fall into a ditch, that somebody will take care of them. Although it should be, it won't be their responsibility. It will be the duty of a civil society. This absence of accountability has to be curtailed.

Every time you turn on the news, you hear about the need for additional funding for these massive government programs. Although it may not solve the entire problem of getting enough dollars into health care, I contend that the amount of fraud and waste that is perpetrated by people who are the scammers and cheats of our society, would more than make-up the need for the additional allocation of money. If we could reduce this massive waste, (that anybody in EMS knows about) it might just be a great start.

A pharmacist who I have known for quite awhile, told me years ago that back in the early 1980's, Michigan imposed a 50 cents per prescription fee to all Medicaid recipients. He told me that after that imposition, he couldn't believe how many of the "junk" prescriptions he no longer filled. So again, my question remains, what do you say to someone who will not spend fifty cents of their own money for medicine they want, but think absolutely nothing of spending more than fifty to one hundred-times that amount of the taxpayers' money for that same medicine?

The answer is that they don't need it. If they did, they would have it. I will not be told by someone with a straight face that I should be concerned about the ability of someone to dig up a dollar or two for needed medicine. By the way, I'm not talking about the senior citizens, or those unfortunate few who are truly disabled and dependent on the care of others for their activities of daily living or for their very survival.

Finally, I think the absolute and undeniable truth to this is that our elected State and Federal government representatives and senators know all of this. I believe they as a whole have known about it for years. I think that because of the fear and dread of being seen as uncaring or not being sympathetic or not understanding the plight of the poor, displaced or disenfranchised; that they fear they may not be re-elected to political office. Therefore, it is much more politically expedient to blame some huge, uncaring, multinational pharmaceutical corporation for exorbitant drug costs. They think they look good to the common citizen when they berate any of the national health insurance companies for spiraling health care premiums.

What a crock!

Political weakness and cowardice is threatening the viability of this nation's ability to continue to deliver quality world-class health care as we have come to know it. Furthermore, I'd like to tell our weak-kneed and gutless politicians that in all of the years I've worked in EMS, I've come to the conclusion that the word "poor" is a relative term.

Sure, we in EMS have seen the poor and the impoverished. We've seen all of the social ills that seem to go hand in hand with poverty. Teenage pregnancy, crime, neglected and abused children, high unemployment, substandard housing and high school dropout rates of fifty percent or more. Each of us in EMS has seen it all. Aside from the neglected and abused children, most of this type of "poor" is a matter of people making poor choices and their attitudes and certainly not by being a victim of random chances or some platitudinous remark made by some hack politician.

At the least, it is in large extent a self-inflicted wound. I believe that if you want to stay poor and never amount to anything in life, what you need to do is become a teenaged, unwed mother and or do illicit and illegal drugs and above all, quit school. All of those are choices we choose to make or choose not to make.

I have seen people who live like pigs. I have seen cockroaches crawling over everything in a house—including their large, wide screen television. I've seen people who smelled so bad that I'm quite sure that soap and hot water were to them like kryptonite was to Superman. I have seen people drink so much alcohol for so long that they literally will lay for days and days in their own ever-increasing excrement.

In short, some people are just content to live in pure, unadulterated filth. It's really just as simple as that. I mean, what else could it possibly be? Your answer might be, "Well Jim, they might be suffering from depression." My answer to that is, "You're right. They might be. I've seen people with real debilitating depression that causes them to not be able to get out of bed in the morning."

That's not who I'm talking about here. I'm talking about those people who don't have anywhere to go and all day to get there. They have no job, no schooling, no responsibility and no goals or expectations for themselves. Who on God's green earth wouldn't be at least a little depressed when faced with a useless and meaningless life such as that?

Unfortunately, too many of the aforementioned people and their ilk, will gladly sit and lay around and wait for someone else to do for them what they as an adult should be fully able, willing and above all expected to do for themselves. And that goes for the wealthy adolescents of our society who have been so insulated that they too know nothing of a hard day's work or personal accountability and responsibility.

I know of a family who was very well-to-do and had several children who were never made accountable to anyone or made responsible for anything. All of them are now adults and not one of them is able to say they are productive, self-sustaining members of society. As far as I know, each of them are solely living off of the inheritance they received when their parents passed away.

I guess as I turn introspective of this thought, my conclusion is that I came from an extremely strong work ethic oriented family. The expectation of daily labor was always present and the fruits thereof were earned and not granted. As a result, I find the slugs of our society annoying. It's not because I'm interested in dictating to people a certain lifestyle. Quite frankly, if you want to live in something that would resemble a pig's sty or a barnyard, so be it. If you don't care to be a productive, gainfully employed member of society, have at it. Just don't expect me to support your parasitic existence. As a hard-working taxpayer, I truly despise subsidizing that way of life.

On the flip side of that, I know that a common household broom is fairly inexpensive. I also know that no one is going to mistake the cost of a bar of soap to that of a bar of gold. I know that a kind word, a loving touch and a caring attitude to your child or children are not only free, but priceless. As a parent and more recently a grandparent, I know that pride cannot be passed on to your children if it's not first practiced by you.

None of these aforementioned things cost much money. So don't look down your nose at me when I look down on some people who call themselves "poor". In today's world, and to this country, the word "poor" is highly arbitrary to say the least.

So for me, there is one undeniable fact that is plain to see for everyone that has an IQ above a stack of pancakes. That one undeniable fact is that unlike anywhere else on this planet, that we, in this country, control our own personal destiny. We can make the choices that will affect us and our children for the rest of our lives. I believe that when you realize that you have that power, you at that moment, cease to be or remain "poor".

If anyone wants to know the definition of being really monetarily poor but not knowing it, let me tell you a brief story. My maternal grandparents lived long before, through, and long after the Great Depression. My mother told me years and years ago how my grandparents lost the farm as the bank foreclosed on their mortgage. She told me how another farmer from a town about thirteen miles away bought their mortgage from the bank for the tidy sum or $4,000.

As a result my mother's family didn't get booted from the farm and thrown into the street. They were able to make payments to the man who now owned the mortgage on the farm. As a matter of record, it took my grandparents more than twenty years to pay off that $4,000 mortgage.

Mom told me that there wasn't any television. There wasn't much time to listen to the radio, and there wasn't much free time for one's own self indulgences. There was an abundance of hard work. From springtime to autumn crops of all kinds were tended. The chickens, pigs, cows, and draft horses had to be cared for and fed each and every day, no matter how cold or hot; or how wet or dry.

Not doing all of those things meant the difference of whether or not you ate that day. I'd be willing to bet that for most people, all of this would be great motivation to get their asses out of bed early every morning and hit the floor running. Long story, short, Mom told me that my grandparents always made sure that she and her siblings were always clean, well fed, worked extraordinarily hard, and were publicly well behaved. She said, she didn't even know they were poor until someone mentioned it one day.

...So getting back to pre-hospital emergency medicine. Let me just say that all of the people who continue to abuse and misuse the emergency services are becoming more of a drain and drag on the system. What's more, they should be called on it through the legislative process.

With the retirement of the Baby-Boomers, the graying of America will not only continue, but accelerate. There will be less of the needed medical services to go around. Healthcare delivery that is already straining to keep up with the demand, is surely going to break. So long as we continue to ignore the facts of a broken system and are reluctant to fix it because of political cowardice, the worse the problem will become. The fact is that there is a bottom to every barrel and I think we are in sight of the bottom of the emergency healthcare barrel. It's almost in a crisis state now. What will it be like in 10, 20 or 30 years from now? Only God knows—and He's not telling.

ACKNOWLEDGMENTS

My editor (who wishes to remain anonymous) was instrumental and totally indispensable in this undertaking. As such, she would remind me when I was becoming too technical while discussing medical terminology and procedures. Through her countless hours of editing and exhausting several red pens, she made the book infinitely better than it ever would have been. Thank you for your tireless efforts.

Attorney at law, Stacy Soper-Stine, was my major legal counsel. She guided me with general legal advice while going through the specific legal hurdles regarding HIPAA. She also assisted me in the chapter structuring of the book and did some specific editing regarding patient anonymity. Thank you so very much.

Many thanks go out to Dr. Robert Kraff, M.D. and to Lori Hellenga, R.N. for their support and for providing me with their medical opinions.

Lastly, I would like to express sincere gratitude to Louise Stine and acknowledge the valuable guidance, encouragement and wise opinions she provided to me.

AUTHOR BIOGRAPHY

James R. Stine Jr. began working as an Emergency Medical Technician (EMT) with the Emergency Medical Services on June 1, 1977; becoming a paramedic in November, 1978. He holds certifications with the American Heart Association and the American Academy of Pediatrics.

He was among the first group of five in southwest Michigan trained to operate an advanced life support ambulance. This training lead him to perform the first-ever advanced life support call while teamed with a basic Emergency Medical Technician (EMT); performing a successful field resuscitation of a cardiac arrest victim.

James, who has answered more than 35,000 emergency calls since he began a career, says this is his life's calling. His debut book is a testament to some of the most memorable calls for help he has answered. He feels this book will open the eyes of those who may not know what paramedics face on a daily basis. In addition, he wants to give tribute to those who answer the calls for help—oftentimes placed in harms way to save others.

He currently lives in southwest Michigan with his wife.

Made in the USA
Monee, IL
24 April 2020